Laryngeal Endoscopy and Voice Therapy

Laryngeal Endoscopy and Voice Therapy

Sue M. Jones

With contributions from
Carrie Garrett

compton
PUBLISHING

Compton Publishing

This edition first published 2016 © 2016 by Compton Publishing Ltd.

Registered office: Compton Publishing Ltd, 30 St. Giles', Oxford, OX1 3LE, UK

Registered company number: 07831037

Editorial offices: 35 East Street, Braunton, EX33 2EA, UK
Web: www.comptonpublishing.co.uk

ISBN 978-1-909082-19-9

A catalogue record for this book is available from the British Library.

Cover design: David Siddall, http://www.davidsiddall.com

Set in Adobe Caslon Pro 12pt by Suart Brown

1 2016

Table of Contents

Acknowledgements

In over thirty years working as a speech and language therapist at the University Hospital of South Manchester in the UK I have worked with some very talented and dedicated colleagues. Some have stayed working in the department and many others have moved on to share their skills elsewhere. In particular, I would like to thank Bev Ashton, Mark Wilson, and Sarah Wallace for their continued professional and personal support.

I have also learned a great deal from laryngologists and voice therapists from other departments who have provided their time and expertise in helping me to improve my knowledge and develop my clinical skills. Above all, I would like to thank Tom Harris and Sara Harris for their encouragement and guidance as I began my foray into voice disorders in the 1980s. Thanks are also due to Paul Carding for guiding me through my MSc in Voice Research.

My expertise in the assessment and management of singers has been greatly enhanced by working with singing teachers and, recently, in collaborating with Carrie Garrett, who comes from a performing/teaching background as well as being a voice therapist. Carrie has co-authored Chapter 3 and Chapter 4 and I am grateful for her enthusiasm and sharing of knowledge.

In addition to Carrie, my colleagues Sara Harris and Jane Shaw kindly agreed to review this manuscript for me and I am indebted to them for their insightful comments.

I am also very grateful to those colleagues who generously allowed me to use their pictures for publication – Stephen Jones, Louise Mattinson, and Leanne Walters. The anatomical illustrations were drawn by Denise de Borde and I am indebted to her for her expertise.

It is only possible to develop as a clinician and be able to achieve your goals if you have colleagues around you who are encouraging and supportive. So thank you to Jude Bibby, Elaine Wilkinson, and Sadie Khwaja, and all those who work or have worked with me in the Speech, Voice and Swallowing Department at University Hospital of South Manchester, UK.

Finally, and most importantly, my husband, Philip H. Jones, Consultant ENT Surgeon – an outstanding laryngologist and teacher – persuaded me that speech and language therapists should perform laryngeal endoscopy and I couldn't have written this book without his encouragement, sharing of knowledge, and support, and my sons, Ben Winstanley and Alex Winstanley, tolerated my trips away from home to further my knowledge without complaint but always welcomed me home.

Preface

I qualified as a Speech and Language Therapist in the UK in 1982. My first job was in a University Teaching Hospital and it brought me into contact with many patients with voice disorders. I loved the work but there were few voice texts available at that time, and much of my therapy was based on instinct and not science. I was a devotee of Daniel Boone's *The Voice and Voice Therapy* as it actually gave some ideas for therapy techniques.

I knew very little about voice disorders but was keen to learn and took the opportunity to sit in as many Ear, Nose, and Throat (ENT) clinics as I could. At that time in our hospital there was no joint voice clinic and the ENT Consultants were not especially interested in voice disorders, but they were patient with me and generous with their time. I cannot say that I learned much about voice disorders, but I did learn a lot about ENT in general.

In the 1980s and 1990s there were countless developments in the knowledge of voice production. Progress was made in the understanding of the vocal fold structure and pathology, perceptual analysis, acoustics, the role of the respiratory system, and laryngeal visualization. There were also advances in the technology available to view the vocal tract, and instrumentation to measure various aspects of voice production. All of a sudden there were numerous texts available on voice disorders and voice therapy.

As interest in voice disorders grew, the approach to their management became more multidisciplinary. Initially, this was joint working between laryngologists and voice therapists, but more recently it has included singing teachers, osteopaths, physiotherapists, and vocal coaches amongst others.

This in turn has resulted in an abundance of voice courses and conferences worldwide, with eminent professionals in all these fields sharing their expertise. I have since had the good fortune to spend time with many of these experts and I thank them for what I have learned in their company.

Throughout my career I have worked at University Hospital of South Manchester, and have been Head of the Speech, Voice and Swallowing Services since 1993. During this time I have had the opportunity to lead the development of the Voice Clinic Services, initially alongside my husband, Philip H. Jones, Consultant ENT Surgeon, and more recently with Sadie Khwaja,

Consultant ENT Surgeon. As well as a running a multidisciplinary voice clinic, voice therapist-led clinics – including those designed specifically for performers – have become a mainstay of our clinical practice. Our aim is always to learn more and develop our skills in order to provide the best clinical services possible for our patients.

The purpose of this book is to act as a practical guide for therapists working in voice clinics and developing voice therapy services. It illustrates how laryngeal endoscopy can help the therapist understand how an individual voice is being produced, both in speech and singing, and how this knowledge can assist in planning therapy. Endoscopic evaluation of the larynx has become an essential part of my clinical practice and I believe it enhances our work as voice therapists.

Sue M. Jones

To my husband, Philip H. Jones, and my sons,
Ben Winstanley and Alex Winstanley.

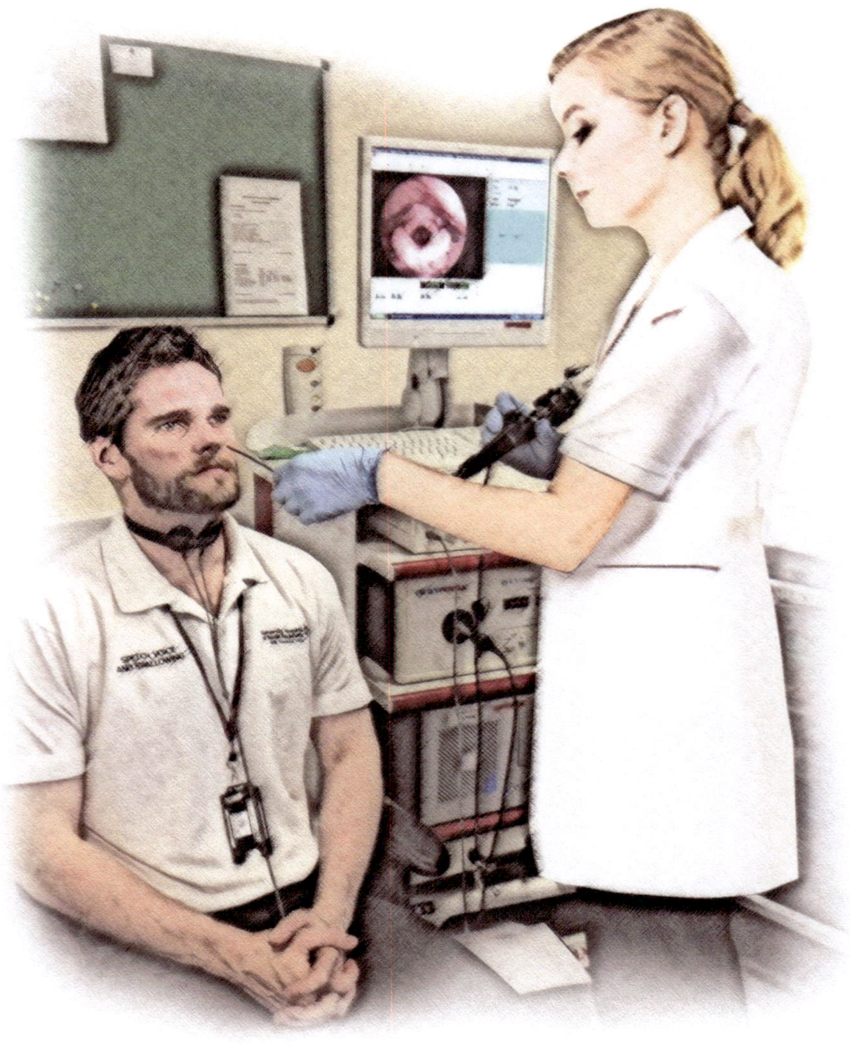

Illustration coutesy of Janine Humphrey

1

Laryngeal Endoscopy

1.1 The developing role of the voice therapist

Until the 1980s, Ear, Nose, and Throat (ENT) surgeons and voice therapists largely worked separately in the management of voice disorders. Patients with voice problems were mostly seen as part of a general ear, nose, and throat caseload by ENT surgeons, primarily in a hospital setting. Laryngeal examinations were initially performed using a mirror and light which gave an adequate view to exclude large lesions, but did not provide any information on how the voice was being produced and, therefore, no guidance for voice therapy. Differential diagnosis was (and remains) the remit of the ENT surgeon and usually, when no vocal fold pathology or neurological abnormality was found on the laryngological examination, the patient would be referred for voice therapy.

Rigid laryngeal mirrors were still the main examination tool in many clinics. Therapists may have seen a brief glimpse of the vocal folds over the shoulder of the ENT surgeon, but no detailed visual assessment of voice production could be made. The introduction of flexible fibre-optic laryngoscopy into ENT clinics enabled the voice therapist to view the vocal tract through the endoscope while the patient was speaking, and this led to a greater understanding of vocal tract physiology and the spoken voice. The development of cameras linked to the endoscopes and of digital videostroboscopy systems allowed joint viewing of the images in real time. This enabled health professionals to discuss examination findings more easily and to provide visual feedback to the patient when discussing management of the voice problem.

In the 1980s joint voice clinics were developed with an increasingly multidisciplinary approach to the assessment and management of voice disorders. One of the earliest of these was established in the UK at Queen Mary's Hospital in

Sidcup, Kent. The inclusion of other professionals, such as an osteopath and a singing teacher, to address the true multidisciplinary nature of the management voice disorders led to this clinic becoming a blueprint for others to follow.[1] This type of multidisciplinary voice clinic still forms the essential foundation for the management of voice disorders and it is imperative for voice therapists to have straightforward access to this type of clinic, even though many other types of voice clinic now exist.

As understanding of the value of laryngeal endoscopy in the assessment of voice disorders from a therapeutic perspective grew, voice therapists began to perform endoscopy themselves. There were no guidelines or professional position statements available at this time, and much of the initial practice was experimental.

In 1994, Karnell published *Videoendoscopy: From Velopharynx to Larynx*,[2] which was the first complete guide specifically for therapists performing endoscopy. This included information on rationale and practical suggestions for passing both flexible and rigid endoscopes.

The American Speech–Language–Hearing Association (ASHA) published a position statement in 1998 concerning the roles of otolaryngologists and speech-language pathologists (SLPs) in the performance and interpretation of strobovideolaryngoscopy, and concluded that SLPs were qualified to use this procedure for the 'purpose of assessing voice production and vocal function'. The position statement is clear that the otolaryngologist is the only professional able to make a medical diagnosis, but that in interdisciplinary settings the diagnostic and functional assessment procedures can be achieved by the combined skills of both professionals.[3] A further position statement was published by ASHA in 2003 outlining the knowledge and skill set required for SLPs for vocal tract visualization and imaging.[4]

There was also recognition by the speech and language therapy (SLT) profession in the UK that endoscopic evaluation of the larynx (EEL) was within the scope of practice for SLTs who were highly specialist in voice disorders, and a position paper was produced by the Royal College of Speech and Language Therapists to provide guidance on the professional clinical context within which EEL was acceptable practice for SLTs. The position paper outlines the context in which SLTs should perform laryngeal endoscopy as well as the competencies, knowledge and skills required. The original position paper was published in 2004, with further revisions in 2008 to reflect continuing developments in practice.[5]

The role of the speech and language therapist in using laryngeal endoscopy is essentially therefore:

- to evaluate vocal function during speech and singing;.
- to trial techniques in order to plan therapy;
- to provide visual feedback to patients in terms of planning therapy; and
- to contribute to confirming the medical diagnosis as part of a multidisciplinary team.

In order to fulfil these roles, the voice therapist will use flexible and/or rigid laryngoscopy with or without , depending on the type of clinic they are working in and the context of the assessment. The voice clinician will need to acquire and maintain the competencies outlined by their professional bodies both in performing and in interpreting the examinations.

1.2 Context of endoscopy in the assessment of clinical voice disorders

Laryngeal endoscopy is clearly only one piece of the jigsaw to be taken into account when assessing voice disorders. Information determined from the case history, auditory-perceptual analysis, observations of posture and breathing, laryngeal palpatory assessment, patient self-report questionnaires, and objective voice analysis all play a key role in reaching a differential diagnosis and determining management. Any programme of voice therapy needs to be based on evidence drawn from all of these elements, and clinicians will tailor their choice of treatment tools based on their overall findings and an individual patient's responsiveness during the rehabilitation programme. Not every patient responds in the same way to each therapy technique[6] and endoscopic evaluation of the larynx can play a key role in determining which techniques most easily achieve the aims of voice therapy for an individual.

1.2.1 Case history

Many authors have published their own case history formats[7–10] with some specifically for professional voice users[11] and clinicians will adapt the best aspects of each of these to inform their own clinical practice. A thorough case history will obtain all the information included in Table 1.1.

Feature	Detail
Personal information	Age, gender, and occupation
Onset of dysphonia	Sudden
	Gradual over days/weeks/months
Progression of dysphonia	Improving/worsening over time
	Variability/consistency
	Episodic/intermittent
	Exacerbating/relieving factors
Patient's main concern	Voice quality/vocal stamina/change in range or volume/ throat pain or discomfort/fear of throat cancer/inability to sing/time off work/comments by friends or family/unconcerned
Voice use	Home/work/social/performing
Previous/ongoing medical history	Diagnosed medical conditions or undiagnosed medical symptoms: respiratory/neurological/gastrointestinal/cardiovascular
	Upper respiratory tract infections: occasional/frequent
	Dysphagia
	Nasal symptoms
	Hearing loss
	Thyroid disorders
	Jaw/dental problems
	Allergies
	Trauma/accidents/injuries
	Surgery: laryngeal/other
	Intubation
	Menstrual cycle
Reflux symptoms	Throat clearing/throat mucus/unpleasant taste in mouth or throat/burning throat
Current medication	Prescribed and non-prescribed
Lifestyle Issues	Smoking: active and passive
	Alcohol consumption
	Recreational drugs
	Environmental irritants
	Weight

Feature	Detail
Vocal care	Hydration
	Diet
	Caffeine intake
Stress and anxiety	Family dynamics
	Major life events
	Emotional reaction to voice problem
	Psychological history
	Current stress levels
	Coping strategies
Previous investigations	Fibre-optic laryngoscopy/rigid laryngoscopy/microlaryngoscopy
	Bronchoscopy/lung function tests
Previous treatment for dysphonia	Medication
	Surgery
	Therapy

Table 1.1: General data required from case history.

There are also a number of structured questionnaires which can be used in addition to the main case history and which can yield further information.

The Vocal Tract Discomfort: Self-Rating Scale[8] allows the patient to rate the frequency and severity of eight throat sensations/symptoms on a five-point scale. These consist of burning, tight, dry, aching, tickling, sore, irritable, and lump in the throat. In addition to providing information for potential therapy intervention, this self-rating scale can act as an outcome measure where vocal tract discomfort is a significant feature of the patient's presentation.

The Reflux Symptom Index (RSI)[12] and Reflux Finding Score (RFS)[13] are also commonly used to determine whether laryngopharyngeal reflux (LPR) plays a significant part in the dysphonia. Diagnosis of LPR is the remit of medical professionals, but the voice therapist who is working independently in a variety of voice clinic settings (see Chapter 2) needs to be aware of the signs and symptoms of LPR, the potential effects on the voice, and the possible management options.

For singers, additional information as detailed in Table 1.2 is also very useful.

Feature	Detail
Specific singing problems	Loss of range – top/mid/low
	Phonation/Pitch breaks
	Vocal stamina during singing
Singing style	Opera/choral/folk/pop/rock/jazz/country/gospel/musical theatre/barbershop/crossover styles
Performance issues	Recent changes in style/repertoire
	Frequency of rehearsal/performance
	Warm-up/cool-down techniques
Type of singing training	Current/previous/ad hoc
Environmental factors	Loud orchestra/band
	Poor amplification/foldback
	Smoky atmospheres/dry ice
	Postural demands during performance
Non-performance related	Socializing after performances
	Travelling schedules
	Diet
	Other vocal demands

Table 1.2: Data specific to singer required from case history.

1.2.2 Perceptual analysis

As clinicians will use information from a variety of sources for assessment and therapy planning, it is impossible to separate what is learned from an EEL examination from the auditory-perceptual evaluation. Madill et al[14] evaluated the consistency, reliability, and agreement made between three experienced clinicians in assessing the effectiveness of training control of the true vocal folds, false vocal folds, and laryngeal height in unimpaired speakers. They found that the judges used their auditory-perceptual skills as well as their visual skills when interpreting the endoscopic examination.

In practice, clinicians will be making an auditory-perceptual analysis of a patient's voice from the moment the initial contact begins. This may be by telephone, in the waiting room, or the clinic room. Other speech disorders such as dysarthria, dysfluency, comprehension, and expressive language difficulties should also be taken into account.[6] Dysphonia can be inconsistent and it is not infrequent for patients to experience an intermittent dysphonia which is not present at the assessment. For both baseline measures and outcome measures, and for planning therapy, a structured auditory-perceptual analysis scheme is essential. The scheme chosen by the clinician will depend on the particular situation. There are various published schemes now commonly in use.

GRBAS scheme

One of the oldest perceptual analysis schemes which is still in common use was developed by The Committee of Phonatory Function Tests of the Japan Society of Logopedics and Phoniatrics. The GRBAS scheme has an overall measure of the severity of dysphonia (Grade) and four parameters (Roughness, Breathiness, Aesthenia, and Strain). The grade and the four parameters are given a value of 0 to 4, with 0 rated as normal, 1 as mild, 2 as moderate, and 3 as severe. The initial publication of the scheme by Hirano in 1982[15] gave little detail on how it should be used. Koschkee and Rammage[10] proposed more detail and specified the 'psychoacoustic' impressions for the characteristics of each parameter. They define these as:

Grade – overall severity or abnormality of the dysphonia;
Roughness – irregular vocal fold vibration;
Breathiness – air leakage through the glottis;
Aesthenia – weak voice; and
Strain – effort and hyperfunction.

The original GRBAS scheme measures laryngeal tone only and, as such, does not assess resonance, pitch, loudness, or many of the other features pertinent to voice production. Dejonckere[16] found the GRBAS scheme to be a reliable perceptual measure of voice and it was recommended by the European Research Group on the Larynx as a tool for clinical and research purposes. Webb *et al.*[17] evaluated the reliability of the three perceptual evaluation schemes most commonly in use at the time (GRBAS, Vocal Profile Analysis Scheme, and Buffalo III Voice Profile) and found that the GRBAS scheme was reliable across all the parameters except strain.

Since then, the scheme has been widely used in studies as a measure of outcome both in voice surgery[18–20] and therapy.[21–24] More recently, the scheme has been used as an outcome measure in assessing vocal quality in head and neck surgery[25,26] and paradoxical vocal fold motion dysfunction.[27] Owing to its limitations, various authors have made additions or alterations to the scheme.

Dejonckere[28] added the parameter of 'instability'. Langeveld[29] added a further six parameters in order to adequately assess the specific vocal aspects of spasmodic dysphonia (aphonia, diplophonia, staccato, tremor, falsetto, and vocal fry).

In 1998, an expert panel of speech and language therapists was commissioned by the British Voice Association to produce a position document on the formal evaluation of voice quality in the UK. The conclusion of this group was that the GRBAS scheme should be used as a minimum standard by all UK SLTs.[30] In 2004, a consensus group was set up by Sue Jones and Paul Carding to discuss the latest developments in vocal perceptual analysis. It was acknowledged that a lack of training courses had resulted in limited dissemination and use of the GRBAS scheme. A training course was developed, based on guidelines and consensus ratings of voices established by this group, and the scheme was extended to include gradings of pitch and loudness.[31,32]

CAPE-V scheme

The Consensus Auditory Perceptual Evaluation of Voice (CAPE-V) was developed by an expert consensus group from the American Speech and Hearing Association. The international group comprised voice scientists, experts in human perception, and speech-language pathologists/therapists. The aim of the consensus group was 'to apply scientific evidence about psychophysical measurement to the clinical practice of judging auditory-perceptual features of voice quality'.[33]

The scheme developed themes already present in the GRBAS system, but expanded to include pitch and loudness. The protocol is administered and scored in a consistent manner. Instead of an ordinal scale, a visual analogue scale is used and the parameters of roughness, breathiness, strain, pitch, and loudness are rated. In addition, there are two further unnamed visual analogue scales included that allow the clinician to rate any additional features which are of note in a particular voice, such as tremor, diplophonia, etc. The rating scale also allows for features to be rated as consistent or intermittent. There are three tasks: sustaining vowels /a/ and /i/ three times for three to five seconds, reading six sentences which are each designed to elicit particular vocal onset patterns, and a period of spontaneous speech. The clinician marks the 100 mm line rating scale for each parameter for each task.

The CAPE-V is more sensitive to changes in auditory-perceptual measures than the GRBAS scheme and is therefore useful to clinicians when measuring outcomes of therapy.

VSPP scheme

The Voice Skills Perceptual Profile was developed by Shewell.[34] It is an auditory-perceptual analysis scheme which assesses in detail the eight parameters of body, breath, channel (vocal tract), phonation, resonance, pitch, loudness, and articulation. There are a different number of key features for the clinician to evaluate within each parameter. Each feature is rated as 0 (no significant features), 1 (mildly significant features), or 2 (markedly significant features).

In total, there are 31 parameters each with a potential rating of 0 to 2, allowing a possible total score of 62. Parameters are judged from conversation and reading. There is also a 'Whole Voice Rating' which is judged by both the client and clinician. This is rated from 0 (no problems) to 3 (severe problems). Because this scheme is so comprehensive it provides a thorough basis for planning therapy, and also offers an overall score which can be used in recording treatment progress.

1.2.3 Musculo-skeletal observations

General observations of habitual posture and breathing are central to the assessment of voice. Postural alignment of the body, neck, jaw, shoulders, and pelvis should be evaluated from both a lateral and anterior viewpoint.[35] Chapman[36] outlines the key factors for good postural alignment in singers and emphasises the importance of 'core stability'. She describes the requirements for flexibility in the abdominal muscles to allow the body to use its own natural elastic recoil during breathing.

Palpatory examination of the neck area is of use to the voice therapist in evaluating the relative positions of the hyoid bone and laryngeal cartilages, as well any inappropriate tension in the extrinsic laryngeal muscles. It can be particularly informative to compare the results of the endoscopic evaluation of the larynx and of the palpatory examination to assess the symmetry of the laryngeal cartilages and the muscles at rest during speaking or singing. Laryngeal muscle tension may be a primary cause of dysphonia or it may occur as a secondary feature due to an individual attempting to compensate for the voice problem, and in doing so increasing tension in the extrinsic and intrinsic laryngeal muscles.[8]

Several authors have described methods and protocols for palpatory assessment of the larynx.[35,37–39] All these authors take care to highlight that this type of assessment should only be carried out by voice therapists who have received instructional training in the procedure. Without a detailed understanding of the anatomy of the head and neck, as well as the palpatory skills taught to perform these protocols, it is possible to cause inappropriate discomfort to patients.

Many authors have described the importance of the assessment of breathing in voice disorders for speakers and singers but breathing techniques remain controversial. Some authors – particularly those who work extensively with singers and actors – recommend breathing techniques as a fundamental element of therapy.[34] Others claim that it is never necessary to work upon breathing.[40] Working upon breathing is likely to be beneficial where the patient's technique is in some way disordered and not conducive to good voice production. It is therefore crucial to assess breathing patterns at rest, during sustained phonation, and during connected speech. These should be evaluated with regard to their impact on an individual's voice and, in particular, patterns of dysfunctional breathing should be noted.

1.2.4 Self-report questionnaires

Self-report questionnaires play a vital part in determining to what extent a patient views their voice problem as affecting their quality of life. They can be used as a basis for deciding with the patient whether or not they wish to attend for therapy at all, and/or as an outcome measure to establish progress. All the self-report questionnaires require a choice to be made from a selection of answers provided. The Voice Handicap Index (VHI),[41] VHI-10,[42] Singing Voice Handicap Index (SVHI),[43] and Voice Symptoms Scale (VoiSS)[44] all have three domains each with a different number of parameters. The Questionnaire of Vocal Performance (QVP),[45] Singing Voice Handicap Index 10 (SVHI-10),[46] Children's Voice Handicap Index 10 (CHVI-10),[47] Vocal Disability Coping Questionnaire (VDCQ),[48] and Voice-Related Quality of Life Scale (V-RQOL)[49] have only one domain, but again vary in the number of their parameters. Scores are calculated, within the domains where applicable, and a total score is reached. Various studies have assessed the validity and reliability of the questionnaires and other studies have tested the correlation between these and perceptual and/or instrumental assessments of voice. Jones and Carding demonstrated that there is good correlation between the severity of dysphonia and the effect on quality of life.[50]

Table 1.3 outlines the questionnaires and their characteristics.

Questionnaire	Number of domains	Number of questions	Parameters for for each question	Total score	Significant score
Questionnaire of Vocal Performance (QVP)	1	12	5 parameters with varying text dependent on the nature of the question, graded in terms of severity of vocal performance	12–60	Not specified
Voice Handicap Index (VHI)	3 (Emotional, functional, physical)	30	0 – Never 1 – Almost never 2 – Sometimes 3 – Almost always 4 – Always	0–120	Score reduction between administrations of 18 or more points
Voice Handicap Index 10 (VHI-10)	3 (Emotional, functional, physical)	10	0 – Never 1 – Almost never 2 – Sometimes 3 – Almost always 4 – Always	0–40	> 11
Singing Voice Handicap Index (SVHI)	3 (Emotional, functional, physical)	36	0 – Never 1 – Almost never 2 – Sometimes 3 – Almost always 4 – Always	0–144	Not specified

Questionnaire	Number of domains	Number of questions	Parameters for for each question	Total score	Significant score
Singing Voice Handicap Index 10 (SVHI-10)	1	10	0 – Never 1 – Almost never 2 – Sometimes 3 – Almost always 4 – Always	0–40	Not specified
Voice-Related Quality of Life Scale (V-QROL)	1	10	1 – None 2 – A small amount 3 – A moderate amount 4 – A lot 5 – Problem is 'as bad as it can be'	10–50	Not specified
Voice Activity and Participation Profile (VAPP)	3 (Perception of voice problem, limitation of, activity, restriction of participation)	28	Visual analogue scale, measured from left of line to give 0–10 for each question: Never ———————— Always	0–280	Not specified
Voice Symptom Scale (VoiSS)	3 (Impairment, emotional, physical)	30	0 – Never 1 – Occasionally 2 – Some of the time 3 – Most of the time 4 – Always	0–120	Not specified

Questionnaire	Number of domains	Number of questions	Parameters for for each question	Total score	Significant score
Vocal Disability Coping Questionnaire (VDCQ)	1	15	0 – Never 1 – Almost never 2 – Sometimes 3 – Quite often 4 – Very often 5 –Always	0–75	Not specified
Children's Voice Handicap Index 10 (CVHI-10)	1	10	0 – Never 1 – Sometimes 2 – Many times 3 –Always	0–30	>4

Table 1.3: Self-report questionnaires

1.2.5 Instrumental voice assessment

Technological development has led to an ever-increasing array of instrumental tools to measure aspects of voice production. These are used in research and have greatly facilitated our understanding of the science of voice production. Equipment to measure pitch, volume, airflow, and vocal fold contact is now widely available for clinicians. Many voice analysis systems can produce a plethora of detail on a wide range of parameters. Baken[51] describes very clearly how a variety of tools can be used and what information can be obtained.

For the practising clinician, however, choosing what is most useful and informative for assessment and planning therapy in a busy clinical setting can be difficult. Instrumentation for clinical purposes needs to be easy to use, meaningful, and reliable. The more recent adoption of relatively inexpensive tablet computers with easy portability and the ability to make high quality and reliable sound recordings has made it easier for voice therapists to use instrumental measures in a clinical environment. There are now a wide range of 'apps' available for analysing voice, and others which can be used in therapy as feedback tools. In daily clinical practice the following measures are often the most easily obtained and useful:

- fundamental frequency (F_0);
- pitch range (both in speech and singing where appropriate);
- jitter (cycle-to-cycle variation in frequency);
- shimmer (cycle-to-cycle variation in amplitude); and
- maximum phonation time.

In an assessment clinic where endoscopic evaluation of the larynx is being performed, instrumental measures can give additional information to aid diagnosis and inform therapy management.

1.3 Anatomy and physiology

Therapists working with voice disorders require extensive knowledge of the anatomy and physiology of the vocal tract. This includes a thorough understanding of the interactions of the vocal tract muscles, as well as the microstructure of the vocal folds. Endoscopic assessments give valuable information with regards to muscle interaction and this is discussed more extensively in Chapter 3 and Chapter 4. Other methods of assessing laryngeal physiology, such as laryngeal palpation, are essential in determining the relationships between positions of the vocal tract structures, including the hyoid bone, thyroid cartilage, and cricoid cartilage.[35,38,39]

1.3.1 Extrinsic laryngeal muscles

The extrinsic laryngeal muscles raise and lower the larynx. They are the suprahyoid and infrahyoid muscles, reflecting their attachments to structures above and below the hyoid bone. The sternothyroid, sternohyoid, and omohyoid muscles are all involved in lowering the larynx. The thyrohyoid, digastric, stylohyoid, mylohyoid, geniohyoid, hyoglossus, and genioglossus raise the larynx.

Figure 1.1 shows the extrinsic muscles of the larynx.

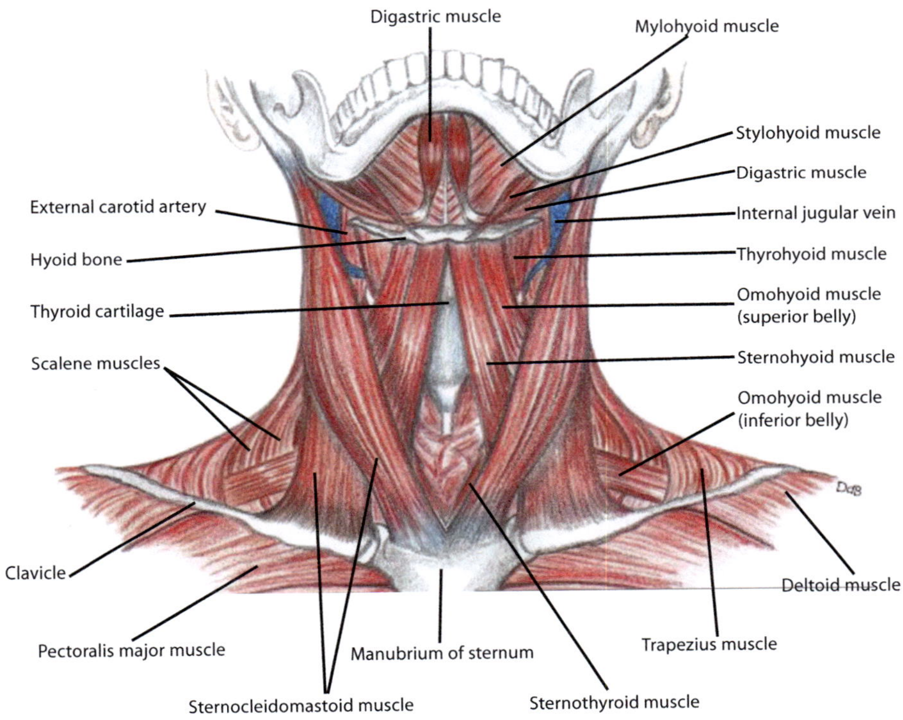

Figure 1.1: Extrinsic muscles of the larynx.

1.3.2 Intrinsic laryngeal muscles

The intrinsic laryngeal muscles are responsible for the abduction and adduction of the vocal folds, degree of vocal fold closure, and the lengthening and tensing of folds to adjust pitch and quality.

In reality, the intrinsic laryngeal muscles largely act together rather than as individual muscles to configure the vocal folds for speech and singing. Table 1.4 outlines the intrinsic laryngeal muscles and their basic functions, and Figure 1.2 shows their positions. It is helpful for voice clinicians to be familiar with texts which describe more extensively the interactions of the intrinsic laryngeal muscles.[52]

Muscle	Function
Posterior crico-arytenoid	Abduction of vocal folds
Lateral crico-arytenoid	Adduction and internal rotation of arytenoid cartilages resulting in 'medial compression' (approximation of the tips of the vocal processes)
Oblique arytenoid	Adduction of vocal folds
Transverse arytenoid	Adduction of vocal folds
Thyroarytenoid	Narrows the laryngeal inlet, shortens the vocal folds
Cricothyroid	Adjustment of vocal fold length

Table 1.4: Intrinsic laryngeal muscles.

The view of the larynx during endoscopy shows the vocal folds from above. Figure 1.3 shows a normal larynx.

1.3.3 Pharyngeal constrictor muscles

It is important to remember the effects of the pharyngeal constrictor muscles in altering the vocal tract configuration during both speech and singing. This is discussed more extensively in Chapter 3 and Chapter 4. There are three pharyngeal constrictor muscles – the inferior, middle, and superior. It is the middle constrictor which plays the greatest role in altering the vocal tract shape, affecting voice projection and singing. Figure 1.4 shows the pharyngeal constrictor muscles.

1.3.4 Microstructure of the vocal fold

The vocal fold is a layered structure. There is a covering layer of epithelium less than 0.1 mm thick. The lamina propria incorporates three layers – superficial, intermediate, and deep. The superficial layer consists mainly of collagen fibres with some elastin fibres, both contained within an interstitial fluid. The intermediate layer has more densely packed elastin fibres. The deep layer contains

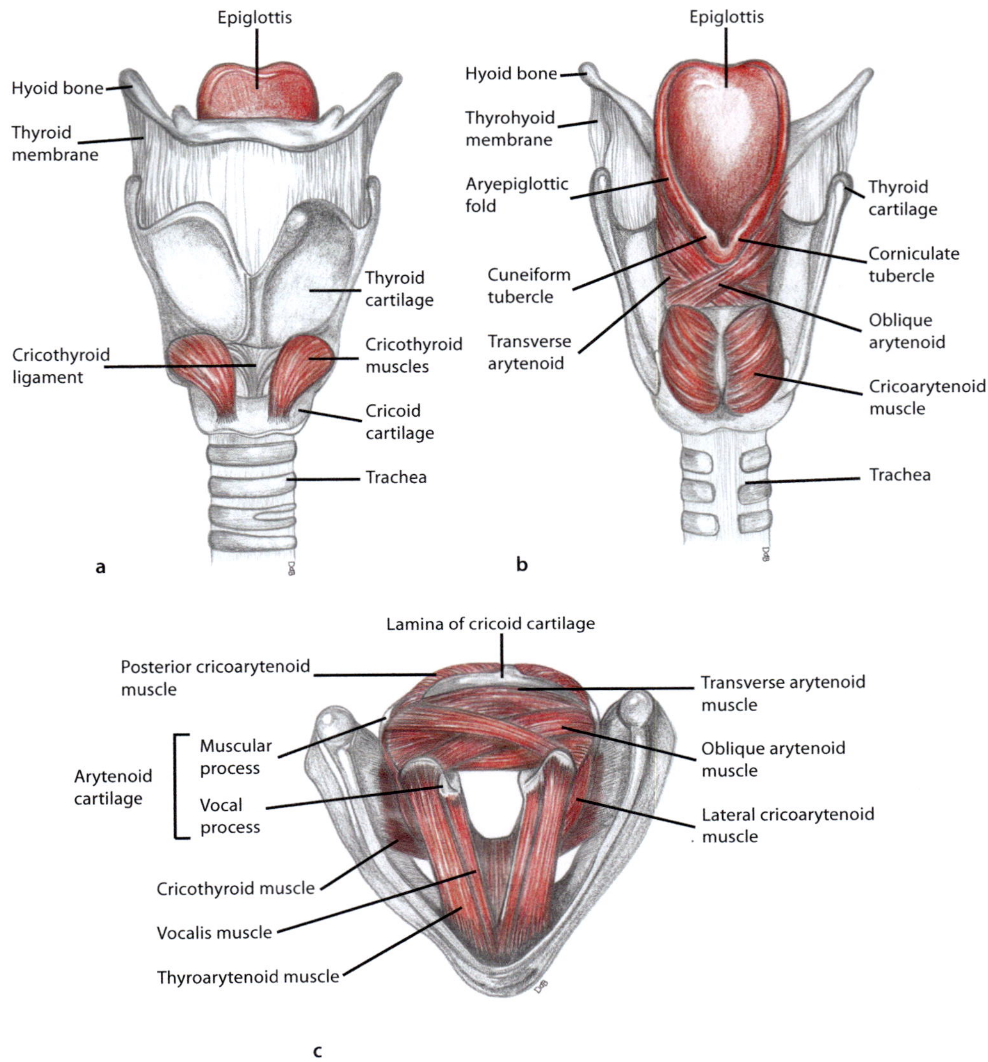

Figure 1.2: Instrinsic muscles of the larynx. **a.** Anterior view. **b.** Posterior view. **c.** Superior view.

mainly collagen fibres. Lateral to the deep layer lies the body of the vocal fold, which contains the vocalis muscle. The vocalis is the medial part of the thyroarytenoid muscle. Referred to by Tom Harris as 'the sophistication of the seemingly simple vocal folds,'[53] it is this complex structure which allows the layered mucosa to move over the body of the vocal fold. Figure 1.5 shows the vocal fold in coronal cross section.

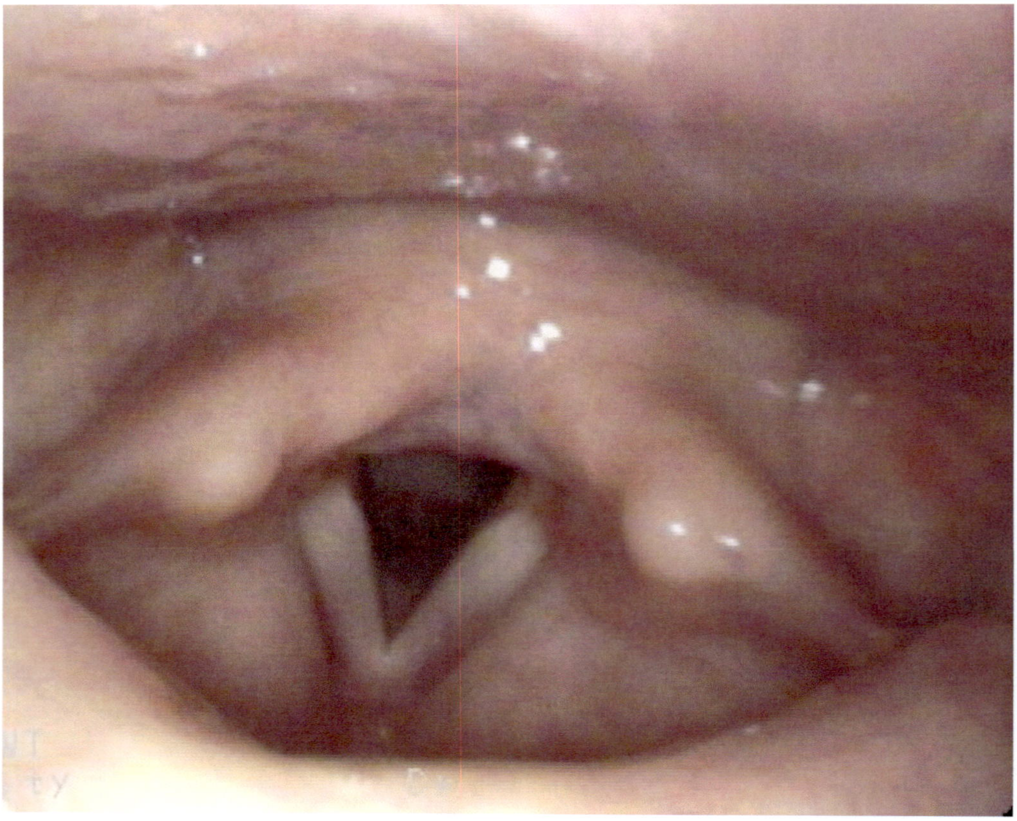

Figure 1.3: Endoscopic view of a normal larynx.

In summary, voice clinicians using laryngeal endoscopy should ensure that they develop an excellent understanding of vocal tract anatomy and physiology. Knowledge can be gained through joint working with laryngologists in daily clinical practice, as well as extensive reading of the current knowledge base.

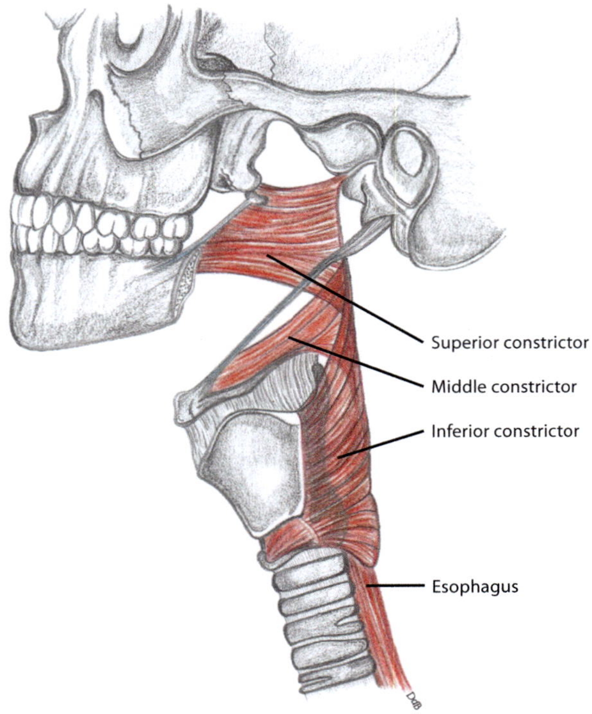

Figure 1.4: Pharyngeal constrictor muscles

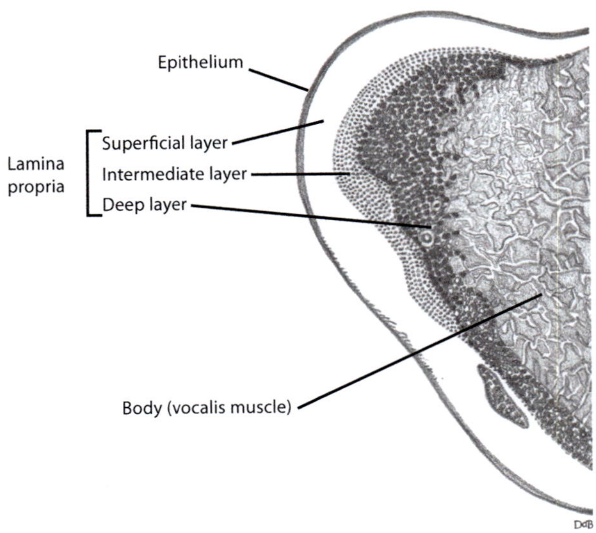

Figure 1.5: Coronal section of the vocal fold

2

Voice Clinics

2.1 Health, safety, and risk assessments

Voice therapists should only perform endoscopic evaluation of the larynx in an appropriate medical setting, with access to other health practitioners in case any unexpected circumstances arise. Complications such as epistaxis and vaso-vagal episodes are extremely uncommon but the clinician needs to be fully aware of the procedures to follow in case of emergencies. Telephone access to a crash team and the presence of resuscitation equipment local to the clinical area are essential.

Individual units will have their own local policies, procedures, and guidelines with regard to health, safety, and risk. Voice clinicians practising laryngeal endoscopy should be also aware of their national and local regulations concerning Control of Substances Hazardous to Health (COSHH),[54] Control of Infection, First Aid, Risk Management, Incident Reporting, and Data Management. In addition, consideration should be given to insurance and liability cover if this is not covered by an employer.

2.2 Equipment and imaging

The earliest visualisation of the human larynx is attributed to Manuel García, a Spanish singing pedagogue. In 1854, inspired by seeing the sun flashing on the window panes of the quadrangle buildings of the Palais-Royal, he bought a dental mirror and a hand mirror. By placing the former against his uvula and using the latter to flash light on its surface, he obtained a view of his own larynx. The use of the laryngeal mirror was taken up by the medical profession world-wide and was still the main instrument for laryngeal examination in the outpatient clinic setting until the development of flexible fibre-optic laryngoscopes in the 1970s.[55]

Flexible fibre-optic laryngoscopes are passed transnasally behind the soft palate into the vocal tract. Views of the vocal tract from the soft palate to the vocal folds can be easily obtained, structures and functions observed, and the interactions of the laryngopharyngeal muscles assessed. This is an ideal examination for assessing voice production from a voice therapy perspective as the patient can speak and sing for long periods without discomfort. More recently, flexible endoscopes with 'chip tip' technology have been developed. These produce higher quality endoscopic images in comparison to the original optical fibrescopes.[56]

Rigid endoscopes are also used for visualizing the larynx. They are available with either a 70 degree or a 90 degree lens. To perform the examination a rigid endoscope is inserted into the back of the mouth. These endoscopes produce a highly magnified view of the larynx with a higher-quality image resolution than that of flexible laryngoscopes. This is essential for detailed examination of the vocal folds and accurate diagnosis of vocal fold lesions. However, their value in assessing the dynamics of the vocal tract is limited as in order to view the larynx the tongue must be pulled forward out of the way. As a result. the patient is only able to produce sustained sound rather than speech. Some patients can only manage this for very short periods and the larynx is glimpsed only briefly, so several attempts need to be made in order to obtain an adequate view for assessment. Others (often singers) can tolerate the examination for long periods and glide on an /i/ vowel very effectively. Furthermore, the positioning of the patient for this examination is not typical of the postures used in speech and singing.

Both flexible and rigid endoscopes can be used with constant light or stroboscopic light. Modern laryngeal examination systems are fitted with both a halogen and xenon light source. The halogen light is constant and steady which does not allow the clinician to view vocal fold vibration patterns, since the vocal folds vibrate at too fast a rate to be perceived by the human eye. However, it is beneficial for viewing the vocal tract structures and functions. The xenon lamp, when triggered, produces a flashing light, affording a stroboscopic view of vocal fold vibration. The timing of the flash is triggered by the fundamental frequency of the voice, which is detected by either a microphone or electroglottograph electrodes placed at the level of the thyroid laminae. The xenon light then flashes at different points within the vibratory cycle, giving the impression that vocal fold movement has been slowed down (an appearance of slow motion) allowing the clinician to see the variations occurring in the movement of the mucosa over the body of the vocal fold. This allows the clinician to identify areas of stiffness and scarring not visible otherwise. It is important to remember that this is just an optical illusion and not a true phenomenon, but stroboscopy does give a valuable perspective in voice assessment and diagnosis.[57]

Various authors[58–63] have pointed out the advantages of the visual feedback that can be given either during or after the examination, should this be welcomed by the patient (which is not always the case). When using visual feedback during the endoscopy, positioning a second linked monitor in the patient's line of view can be very useful.

There are many companies manufacturing flexible and rigid laryngeal endoscopes, as well as laryngeal examination stacks which enable digital recording, analysis, database facilities, and report production. Other benefits of this equipment include reviewing recordings in slow motion, and dual screen comparison between current and previous laryngeal examinations. Technology is constantly developing and the voice therapist needs to judge what may be the best equipment for the purposes of laryngeal endoscopy in relation to voice therapy. Relatively new techniques such as narrow band imaging,[64] videokymography,[65] and high speed photography[66] may well prove to be tools for the future for the voice therapist, although they are not currently used in everyday practice. This book considers the equipment in common use in clinical settings and how the voice therapist can make best use of this.

2.3 Clinic types

There are several different types of voice clinic in which voice therapists perform endoscopic evaluation of the larynx. Some are primarily diagnostic, others are orientated more towards therapy planning. More recently, therapists have begun to perform endoscopy during voice surgery procedures carried out in a day case setting under local anaesthesia. The various types of clinic are outlined below.

2.3.1 Joint voice clinic/combined voice clinic

Patients are assessed in a multidisciplinary clinic with several professionals offering their expertise in reaching a diagnosis and planning management. The core team will be a laryngologist and a voice therapist with extensive experience in voice disorders. Other professionals who may attend on a regular or ad hoc basis as part of the extended team are a singing teacher, vocal coach, osteopath, psychologist, neurologist, and respiratory physician. This is an ideal setting for making a differential diagnosis and for management planning as clinicians can each bring their expertise to the multifactorial aspects of voice disorders.[1]

The overall responsibility for patient diagnosis and care remains with the consultant laryngologist.

2.3.2 Parallel voice therapist-led voice clinic

This type of clinic is led by a voice therapist alongside another clinic run by the laryngologist (which may be non-voice related). Patients are triaged from referral letters, using strict selection criteria. Patient selection is aimed at those most likely to have non-organic voice disorders; any patients with 'red-flag' indicators, such as smoking and complex medical co-morbidities, should be excluded and seen in the joint clinic. Although the voice therapist will work independently, taking a case history, performing EEL, and perceptual/instrumental/palpatory measures, all images will be discussed with the consultant laryngologist and she or he will retain overall responsibility for patient diagnosis and care. In some parallel clinics, post-operative patients, where histology has shown a lesion to be benign, are also reviewed as they may require voice therapy as part of their rehabilitation.

2.3.3 Voice therapy assessment clinic

Not all voice referrals for voice therapy will come through a joint voice clinic. Many will be referred from general ENT clinics or assessment units based at general practitioner surgeries. Others may have been seen in other hospitals for voice assessment before being passed on to local services. In most instances, patients referred in these ways will have had no video imaging and no access to stroboscopy. The therapist will not have had the opportunity to view the larynx or to assess the potential impact of voice therapy. Voice therapists may therefore wish to examine the vocal tract, including stroboscopy where available, in order to establish a more detailed understanding of how an individual is producing their voice and to trial various therapy techniques. This aids therapy planning and patient compliance with treatment. On occasions, experienced voice therapists will identify abnormalities not detected in previous examinations and will need to bring this to the attention of the laryngologist in the joint clinic setting in a timely manner. Some voice therapy clinics may be specifically orientated towards a particular patient group, such as performers, and be attended by other relevant professionals, such as singing or vocal coaches.

2.3.4 Laryngeal intervention clinic

This is a multidisciplinary clinic based in an out-patient or theatre setting which delivers surgical laryngeal interventions. Such interventions are performed under endoscopic view and it is the role of the voice therapist to perform the endoscopy, providing advice on the perceptual quality of the voice to the laryngologist during the procedure, and delivering post-operative care and follow-up to the patient.

2.4 Knowledge and skills

In order to perform any of these roles a high level of expertise is required. Laeeq and colleagues[67] evaluated the number of attempts by medical students to become competent in passing a flexible nasendoscope and found that the mean was 6 with a range of 2–17. However, the study involved the participants using a mannequin rather than patients in a clinical setting. The voice therapy clinician needs to become proficient at both passing the flexible and rigid endoscopes and interpreting the images seen. The latter is a skill which takes many years to acquire at an expert level, and clinicians who are in training to be specialists in voice disorders benefit from attending voice clinics regularly in order to become familiar with endoscopic footage.

The particular knowledge and skills acquired by the voice therapist should be at an advanced clinical standard. Both the American Speech–Language–Hearing Association and Royal College of Speech and Language Therapists have defined these skill sets.[4,5]

2.4.1 Knowledge required

- Normal and abnormal nasal, velopharyngeal and laryngeal anatomy and physiology.
- Physiology of normal and abnormal voice production.
- Awareness of health and safety and risk assessments, including endoscope decontamination.
- Awareness of local policies and procedures appertaining to EEL.
- Understanding of requirement to practice EEL within professional guidelines.

- EEL protocols and their rationale.
- Principles and techniques of voice therapy.
- Effects of medication.

2.4.2 Skills required

- Choice of appropriate type of EEL procedure (i.e. flexible or rigid).
- Putting clients at ease, with adequate explanations of the purpose and nature of the examinations.
- Administering topical nasal anaesthesia where appropriate.
- Passing flexible and rigid endoscopes and obtaining high quality images without causing discomfort to the patient.
- Interpretation of phonatory physiology patterns and their significance in making a voice therapy diagnosis and planning therapy.
- Selection of appropriate therapy techniques to trial during the endoscopic procedure.
- Making an accurate voice therapy differential diagnosis.
- Organization, storage, and retrieval of EEL data for audit, treatment effectiveness and legal purposes.
- Provision of appropriate and informative visual and verbal feedback to patients.
- Judgement as to when further medical/surgical opinion should be sought.

2.5 Practical endoscopy techniques

2.5.1 Topical nasal anaesthesia: the evidence base

Practice with regard to routine use of topical nasal anaesthesia, vasoconstrictors, and lubricating agents in the setting of an outpatient clinic is inconsistent. Various studies have investigated the effectiveness of these and, although a Cochrane review in 2011[68] concluded that there did not appear to be good evidence for routine use of a topical spray before laryngeal endoscopy, they also observed that many of the studies had methodological problems or inadequate sample sizes to draw satisfactory conclusions. Other authors recommend the use of topical nasal anaesthesia for all laryngeal examinations[69] and it is still widely used in clinical practice.

Frosh et al[70] when comparing the use of lidocaine, saline, and no anaesthesia, found that the lidocaine increased the unpleasantness experienced by the patient during the procedure and recommended that topical anaesthesia should not be used prior to laryngeal endoscopy.

Sadek et al[71] in comparing the effects of three types of topical anaesthesia with no anaesthesia concluded that vasoconstrictor effect rather than the local anaesthetic itself was a key factor in reducing discomfort and improving tolerance during laryngeal endoscopy. These authors also concluded that not using any nasal preparations led to the experience of severe symptoms.

Smith et al[72] compared the use of cocaine and cophenylcaine (5% lidocaine and 0.5% phenylephrine solution) during endoscopy. Cocaine has been used traditionally in ENT OP settings but their findings showed that cophenylcaine was equally effective and a less toxic option.

Cain et al[73] carried out a double-blind randomized controlled trial on 90 patients. The groups were randomized to receivie cophenylcaine spray, a placebo spray, or no nasal preparation. The primary outcome measures used were pain and overall discomfort. The authors concluded that there were no significant differences on these measures between any of the three groups and therefore that the routine use of topical nasal preparation before nasendoscopy could be discontinued.

Johnson et al[74] performed transnasal fibre-optic laryngoscopy on 15 patients, each on three separate occasions. The fifteen subjects received one of 4% cocaine, 0.05% oxymetazoline, or saline to both nasal cavities. Each subject received a different preparation on each of their three examinations. The study's conclusions were that a topical anaesthesia such as cocaine was justified as it significantly reduced patient discomfort during the procedure.

Georgalas et al[75] performed a prospective double-blind randomised controlled trial on 98 patients in their UK clinic and found that there was no significant difference in pain or the overall discomfort experienced between those receiving cophenylcaine spray and those receiving a saline placebo. The sensation of bad taste, however, was significantly worse in the cophenylcaine group.

Douglas et al[76] in comparing the relative effectiveness of cophenylcaine and lignocaine during rigid nasal endoscopy concluded that the two sprays produced similar levels of local anaesthesia but the vasoconstrictor effect of the cophenylcaine improved the ease of passing the endoscope and image quality for the practitioner.

Bourolias et al[77] compared the use of 2% tetracaine solution and 10% lidocaine spray applied to each nasal cavity on microsponges for ten minutes prior to laryngoscopy. Results showed that the participants who received tetracaine experienced significantly lower nasal discomfort, with no complications or side effects.

Shrestha and Amatya[78] found that there was no benefit to using topical nasal anaesthesia before flexible nasopharyngolaryngoscopy in comparison to a saline spray in terms of patients nasal pain, throat discomfort, bad taste, feeling of nausea, or overall discomfort.

Evidence base for use in terms of discomfort

Mahrous et al[79] performed a study to determine whether passing the nasendoscope above or below the inferior turbinate made a difference to patient discomfort. Discomfort was assessed using a visual analogue scale. No significant difference in discomfort was found between the two groups. This study did not use topical nasal anaesthesia, but did use a lubricant gel for all study participants.

Hu et al[80] performed a prospective cohort study on 102 participants with laryngeal pathology to determine whether oral topical anaesthesia administered prior to rigid laryngoscopy had any effect on vocal quality. Acoustic and perceptual measures were used to determine vocal change. The authors concluded that the use of oral anaesthesia did not change vocal quality and supported the view that this should be used where the clinician feels it is indicated.

Jacobs and Kenny[81] examined the acoustic and perceptual effects of topical anaesthesia during fibre-optic laryngoscopy against a control condition in the singing voices of ten professional sopranos. The results showed that the presence of anaesthetic and the laryngoscope did not significantly affect their singing.

Pothier et al[82] found that endoscope insertion and image quality were improved (as reported by the endoscopist) when using water rather than a standard lubricant such as K-Y Jelly. There was no reported difference in the unpleasantness felt by the patient.

Use of topical nasal anaesthesia in the voice therapist's clinical practice

All voice clinicians will come across patients who are very anxious with the thought of the endoscopy procedure and who benefit psychologically from a topical anaesthesia. Other patients will have had a bad experience from a previous examination and may find the use of the anaesthesia reassuring. Preparing the patient for the examination is an important part of obtaining the best quality images and learning as much as possible about their voice production from the examination. An anxious patient will not be able to tolerate the procedure as easily and therefore will be less likely to be able to co-operate with the vocal tasks required. Laryngeal endoscopy protocols for voice therapy tend to take much longer than a typical ENT examination with the endoscope often in place for between three and six minutes.

Conversely, some patients prefer to be examined without the topical nasal spray and cope very well with a long examination. It is the clinician's skill and judgement along with patient choice that are required to decide best practice for each individual.

Use of a lubricating gel, especially with patients who have not had a topical anaesthetic to the nose, can be beneficial in helping to pass the endoscope smoothly through the nasal passage. However if the gel mists the distal end of the scope it can obscure the view and can be difficult to remove without withdrawing and reinserting the scope.

Clinicians' practice varies in how the anaesthesia is administered. Some clinicians spray topical nasal anaesthesia – several puffs into both nostrils; others spray the nostril which the patient or clinician feels is most patent. The latter is usually because the topical anaesthesia tastes bitter and spraying one nostril can be less uncomfortable. There is no evidence to suggest any one method is superior to another in terms of patient comfort, ease of passing the endoscope, or image quality.

In the United Kingdom, where voice therapists apply a topical nasal anaesthesia prior to laryngeal endoscopy, a Patient Group Direction (PGD) needs to be developed in conjunction with the pharmacy department, and a written record kept of all clinicians within the organization who are trained in its administration.[83]

Patient Group Directions (PGDs) should be agreed locally. They should include:

- the clinical condition to which the PGD applies;
- inclusion/exclusion criteria;
- actions to take if the patient is excluded from or declines to have the medicine (this is not of such concern in laryngeal endoscopy as the procedure can be performed without topical nasal anaesthesia);
- staff qualifications (registered speech and language therapist/pathologist);
- additional requirements:

  - appropriate specialist training as detailed in the Royal College of Speech and Language Therapists 'Endoscopy for Voice Disordered Patients'[84] or the American Speech and Hearing Association 'Knowledge and Skills for Speech-Language Pathologists with respect to vocal tract visualization and imaging',[4]
  - training in resuscitation procedures, updated in line with local policies, and
  - local training on the administration of topical nasal anaesthesia;
- details of the drug name, form, strength, dosage, frequency, duration of treatment, and side effects; and
- details of what to do if an adverse event occurs, advice to be given to patient/carer, and a follow-up contact for any patient concerns.

2.5.2 Patient preparation and endoscope techniques

Clinic set-up

If the voice therapist is working in a voice clinic independently, it is essential to operate the clinic with an assistant. The role of the assistant is primarily to liaise with patients before the examination, prepare and operate the examination equipment during the procedure, and to ensure data is obtained and stored appropriately. It is also necessary to have an assistant in the clinic in case the patient becomes unwell or distressed during the procedure. This role can be fulfilled by a nurse, technical instructor, or therapy assistant, providing they have the requisite knowledge and skills. In a multidisciplinary clinic this role is not as vital as these tasks can be taken on by other members of the team, but the presence of an assistant can still be very useful as it allows the other professionals to concentrate on their own responsibilities. The assistant should have a thorough knowledge of how the examination equipment is operated, know how to handle flexible and rigid endoscopes safely, and have the ability to put patients at their ease by explaining the clinic procedures.

Obtaining good quality images during the EEL is essential. Good planning and careful patient preparation are fundamental to the success of the procedure.

The examination system needs to be set and up ready. Before beginning the procedure the endoscope and camera should be assembled, on the correct setting, and focussed. Most of the digital videostroboscopy systems in clinical use have extensive settings and it is distracting if frequent alterations are made during the endoscopy. The endoscopist should be comfortable and able to reach any foot pedals required during the process.

The patient should be appraised of what will happen during the procedure and approximately how long it is likely to take. When performing rigid laryngeal endoscopy, patients should be informed they will be asked to produce a sustained /i/ vowel at varying pitches and that it is the attempt at the /i/ rather than the resulting sound that is important. With flexible laryngeal endoscopy it is helpful to state that they will be asked to carry out a number of vocal tasks and details of the tasks provided. If the patient has problems with their singing voice and the Singer's Protocol (see Chapter 4) is being used, it is essential to ensure they have chosen the songs they plan to sing before the procedure commences as many find themselves unable to remember any of their repertoire once the EEL procedure has begun.

Flexible laryngeal endoscopy

The patient should be seated at the correct height using an adjustable chair so that the endoscopist can perform the examination comfortably without back or arm strain. If the patient's feet do not reach the floor a foot rest should be provided.

Ask the patient to sit facing forwards with uncrossed legs, both slightly over to one side and stand next to him/her on the opposite side. Their body should not be twisted. Stand on the same side as the endoscope will be inserted. The endoscopist standing between or over the patient's legs can be personally discomforting for both parties.

Ensure the patient's head is in an upright position, not falling backwards or slouching forwards, as this will lead to poor patient positioning in the chair, causing the endoscopist to lean further forwards or backwards and as a result poor views will be obtained. These positions are also not conducive to obtaining the best vocal quality in either speech or singing.

Ask the patient to relax their shoulders as much as possible and to keep the torso upright, as this will produce a better overall position of the head and neck during the examination.

Explain to the patient that they will be able to breathe, cough, swallow, and speak normally during the flexible examination.

Karnell[2] advocates a standing position for singers during flexible laryngeal endoscopy as it is easier to sing in this position. The ease or difficulty of this will be determined by the relative heights of the patient and examiner and may require a steady, safe platform for the endoscopist to use. Clinical experience indicates that the larynx of a highly-trained pop singer can be difficult to keep in view while she or he is performing very athletic styles such as 'belt' in a standing position. Figure 2.1 and Figure 2.2 illustrate good and bad positioning for flexible laryngeal endoscopy.

Inserting the flexible endoscope

When passing the endoscope through the nasal passage and into the vocal tract, the therapist may encounter uncommon or abnormal nasal and/or vocal tract anatomy. Figure 2.3 illustrates some of the most commonly observed.

The endoscope should be inserted into the more patent nasal passage. This can be initially checked by asking the patient which nostril is easier to breathe through. If she or he is unsure, the clinician should close each nostril in turn whilst asking the patient to breathe through the nose. This will often determine any difference in patency between the two nostrils. Another option is to insert the endoscope just into the front of the nasal passages on each side and note whether there is any observable difference between the two.

Once inserted into the nares, the endoscope can be passed either along the floor of the nasal passage under the inferior turbinate or through the middle meatus between the inferior and middle turbinates. McFarlane and Lavorato[62] favour passing the endoscope along the floor of the nose whereas Karnell,[2] Harris,[1] and Koufman[69] all recommend the latter approach, as the endoscope is likely to rest further away from the superior surface of the soft palate once fully inserted and therefore have a lesser effect on the elevation of the soft palate during the assessment. The selected route through the nasal passage will be influenced by the individual's nasal anatomy. A deviated nasal septum, septal spur, septal perforation, nasal polyps, and/or swollen nasal turbinates may all impede easy passage through the nose. Use of a vasonconstrictor with or without topical anaesthesia will reduce nasal turbinate swelling thereby reducing patient discomfort. Figure 2.4 illustrates the alternative insertion routes.

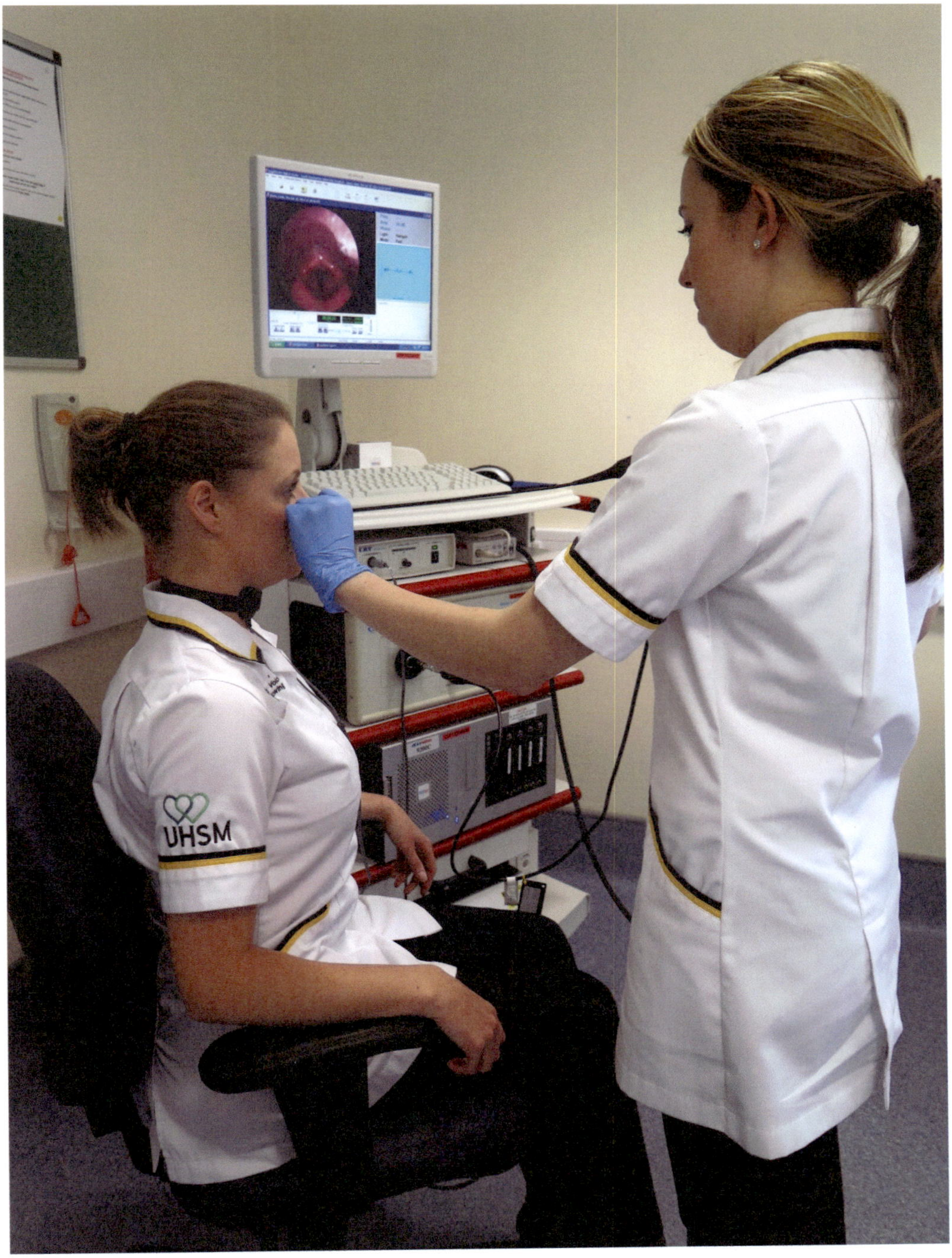

Figure 2.1: Good positioning for flexible endoscopic examination.

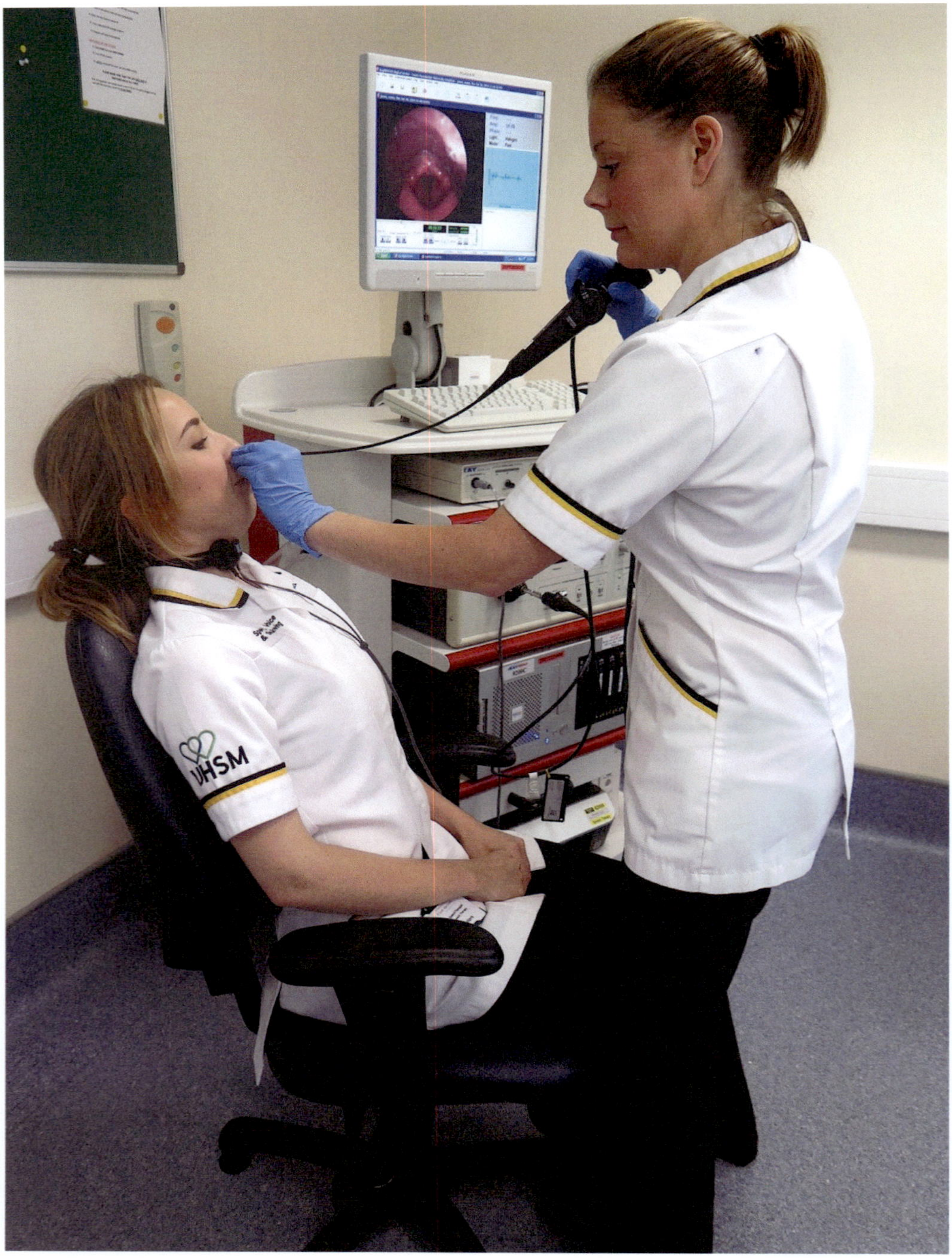

Figure 2.2: Poor positioning for flexible endoscopic examination.

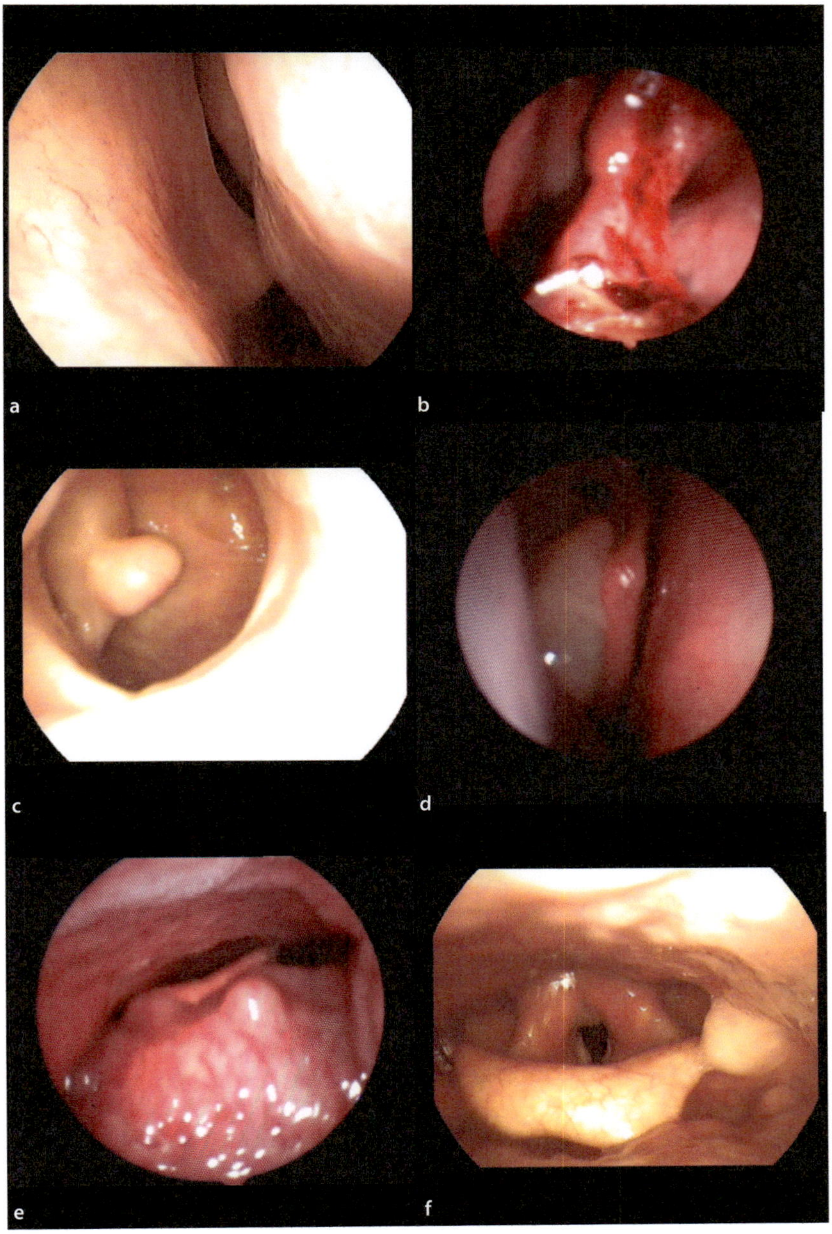

Figure 2.3: Abnormal nasal anatomy. **a.** Nasal septal spur. **b.** Absent nasal septum. **c.** Nasal cyst. **d.** Nasal polyp. **e.** Base of tongue cyst. **f.** Vallecula cyst.

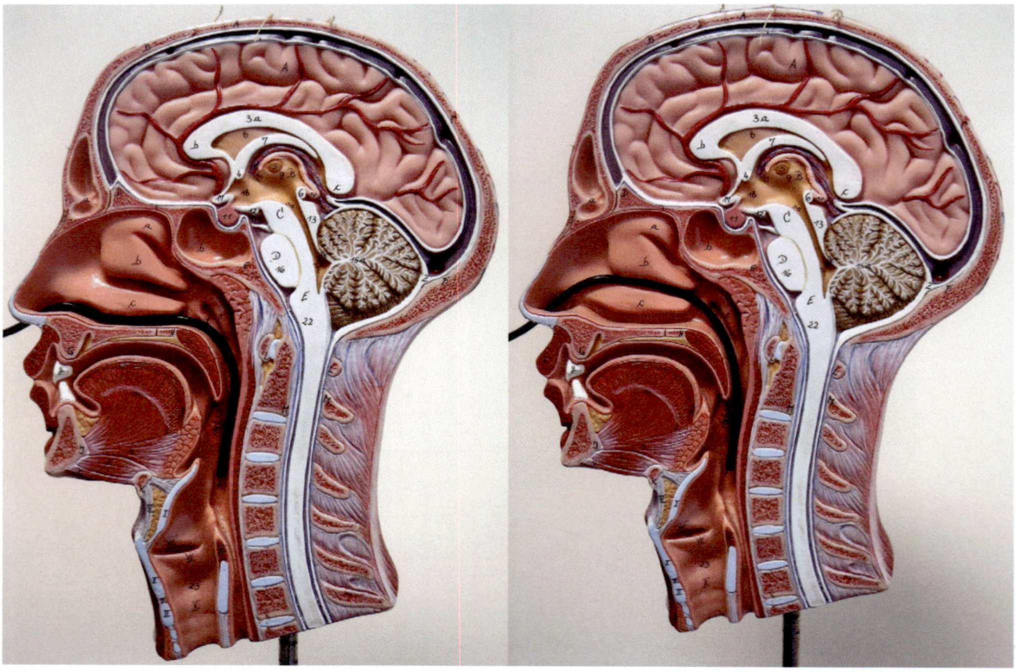

Figure 2.4: Endoscope insertion routes. **a.** positioning along floor of nose. **b.** positioning through the middle meatus

Passing the flexible endoscope

1. Keep the tip of the endoscope straight prior to insertion.
2. Insert into the most patent nostril either along the floor of the nose or through the middle meatus, depending upon the nasal anatomy.
3. Hold the distal end of the endoscope with the finger (or finger and thumb) resting gently on the patient's nose. Do not press too firmly as this causes discomfort.
4. Avoid twisting the endoscope during insertion – keep the arm straight.
5. Push gently but steadily forwards.
6. Aim towards the posterior pharyngeal wall. Light will be reflected from this area.
7. Once in the postnasal space, turn the distal end of the scope towards the larynx using the endoscope lever. Head for 'blackness' ensuring the endoscope is in space. If the image becomes pink or white the endoscope is touching tissue and it will be necessary to retract the scope to the postnasal space. If the velopharyngeal port is closed ask the patient to 'close the mouth and breathe through the nose' to open it. This is more common in highly anxious patients.

8. Push gently towards the larynx until the vocal folds come into view.
9. Difficulties in obtaining a good view may be caused by any of the following:
   - tongue backing: ask the patient to protrude the tongue;
   - pharyngeal tension: ask the patient to yawn gently; or
   - omega epiglottis shape: ask the patient to protrude the tongue and sigh whilst manipulating the distal end of scope over epiglottis using the scope lever.
10. Keep the endoscope in the centre of the vocal tract above the epiglottis until the patient is comfortably settled before proceeding with the voice assessment protocol.
11. For a closer view of the vocal folds and to assess vibratory characteristics during stroboscopy, advance the endoscope towards the laryngeal vestibule, using the endoscope lever to change the angle at the scope tip. To obtain the best view, aim to remain in the centre of the vocal tract.
12. If the central view is lost, use both hands to move the scope laterally and the lever to readjust the scope angle.
13. If the endoscope image becomes unclear owing to mucus secretions, these can usually be cleared by asking the patient to swallow. Sometimes this will need to be repeated several times before the lens clears.

Rigid laryngeal endoscopy

As with flexible endoscopy, the patient should be seated at the correct height (use an adjustable chair) so the endoscopist can perform the examination comfortably without back or arm strain. Some clinicians prefer to stand whilst performing this procedure whilst others obtain a better image from a seated position. Obtaining the best quality image is the key factor and there is no right or wrong way.

Topical anaesthesia may be sprayed onto the soft palate and posterior pharyngeal wall in order to desensitize the area and minimise any gag reflex. Some patients will tolerate rigid laryngeal endoscopy without anaesthesia but it is generally accepted that this form of examination can be more challenging for patients and can often only be managed for short periods of time.[2] Therefore the rigid scope may need to be inserted on several occasions to obtain adequate views or sufficient data to allow accurate diagnosis and informed management. Patient position and examiner skill play a key part in the success of the procedure.

The rigid scope is inserted through the oral cavity towards, but not touching, the posterior pharyngeal wall. The angle of insertion required to acquire a good image will depend on whether a 70 degree or 90 degree rigid endoscope is being used. The 90 degree rigid scope will require the patient to sit in a more upright position. When using a 70 degree scope the patient should bend forwards slightly from the waist and elevate the jaw. The scope should be held as steadily as possible. Some examiners prefer to stabilize the scope by placing it on the patient's upper teeth,[2] others advocate avoiding contact with the oral cavity if possible.[86] Tongue anchoring is often used, where the patient's tongue is extended out of the mouth and held (by themselves or the examiner with a piece of gauze) whilst the rigid scope is inserted. Morrison and Rammage report that placing the rigid endoscope in a lateral position in the mouth and rotating the camera at its attachment to the scope to correct the angle produces a good view.[87]

The examination can be more difficult if the patient has a long uvula which needs to be lifted out of the way or a particularly sensitive gag reflex. Asking the patient to breathe through their mouth will lift the soft palate and may make it easier to obtain good views. As the endoscope is inserted the patient's breath may cause the lens to fog. To avoid this, a few drops of a demisting agent can be used on the end of the scope prior to insertion. Another method of to prevent fogging of the lens is to insert it into hot water just prior to the procedure. Alternatively, wiping the rigid endoscope on the buccal/tongue mucosa or on the gauze being used to hold the patient's tongue may work equally well.

The aim of this examination is to achieve a high quality image of the full length of the vocal folds. Better views of the anterior commissure can be obtained by asking the patient to phonate on a sustained /i/ vowel. Once good views have been obtained the rigid endoscopic protocol can be followed. Figure 2.5 shows the rigid endoscope procedure.

2.6 Laryngeal anatomy

If a voice therapist is performing EEL independently and not in a joint voice clinic setting, this will usually be to assess the potential effects of voice therapy techniques. Patients will most often have undergone an examination by an ENT surgeon previously to exclude laryngeal abnormalities. However, as clinical practice has developed, highly-experienced voice therapists have also began to run assessment clinics independently where it is safe practice to do so and to assess

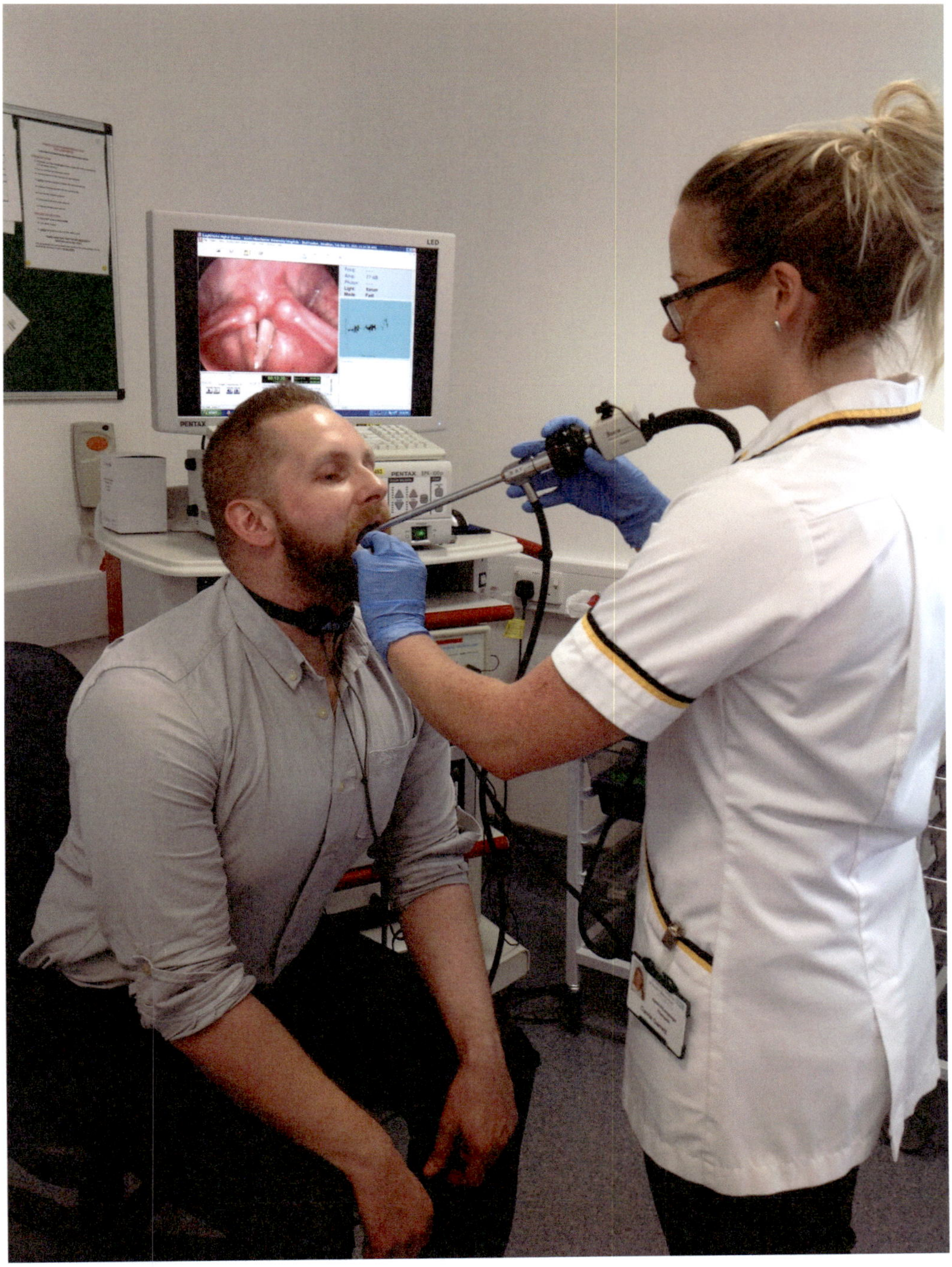

Figure 2.5: Performing rigid laryngeal endoscopy.

patients using strict selection criteria (see Chapter 2). It is therefore essential for the voice therapist practising in these circumstances to have an excellent knowledge of abnormal laryngeal structures. Many appropriate texts are available for the voice clinician such as *Atlas of Laryngoscopy* by Sataloff et al.,[85] which details both common and rare laryngeal conditions. All such abnormalities must be brought to the attention of the consultant laryngologist.

Figure 2.6 illustrates some of the most common benign laryngeal conditions which the voice therapist may encounter.

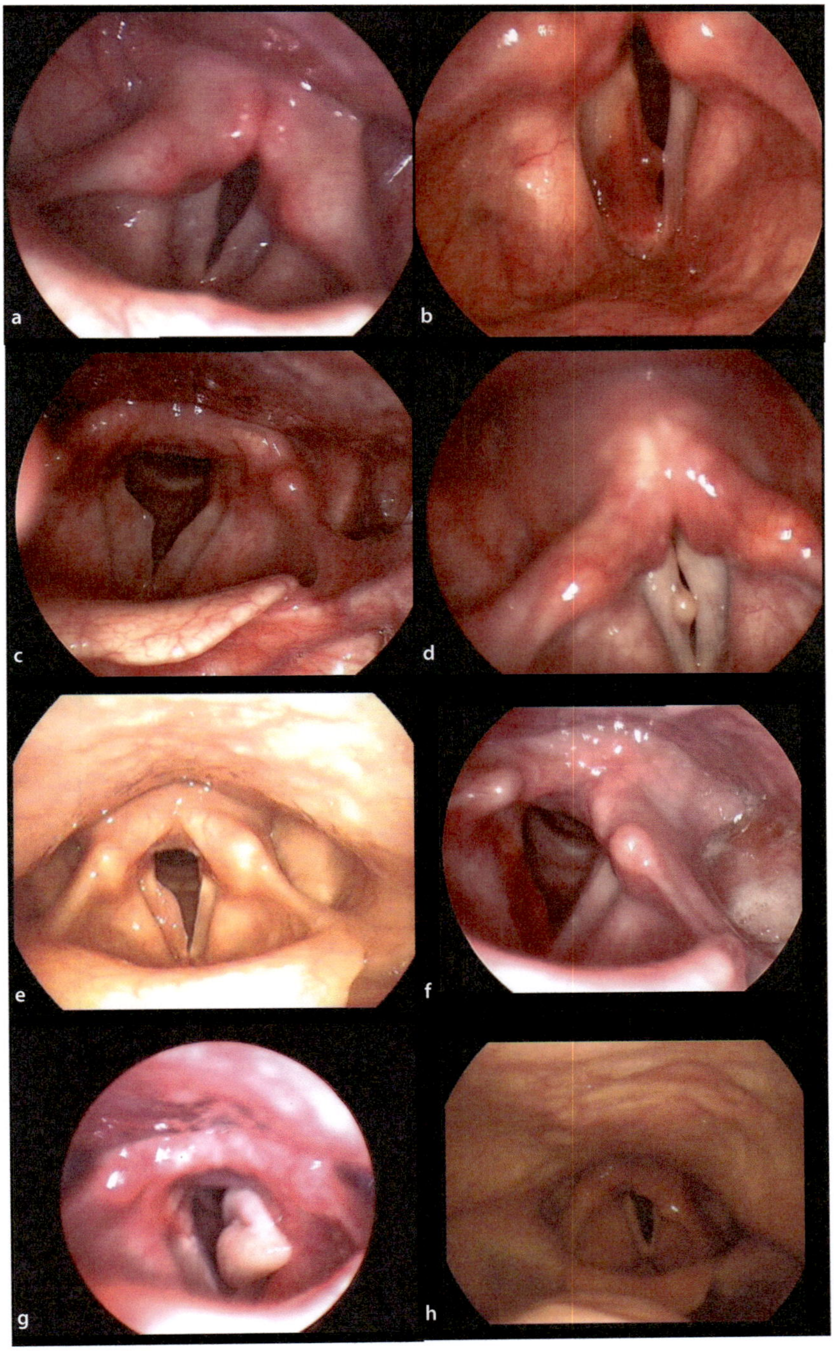

Figure 2.6: Common laryngeal conditions. **a**. Nodules. **b**. Polyp with haemorrhage. **c**. Polypoidal degeneration. **d**. Vocal fold cyst. **e**. Papilloma. **f.** Vocal fold haemorrhage. **g**. Arytenoid granuloma. **h**. Left vocal fold palsy.

3

Assessment Protocol for the Spoken Voice

Sue Jones and Carrie Garrett

There are a number of published protocols or suggested datasets with a structured approach to follow during endoscopic evaluation of the larynx. Most of these are oriented towards using stroboscopy for evaluation and/or measurement of structure and identifying abnormalities, rather than assessment of the function of the whole vocal tract.[86,88–92] For differential diagnosis of subtle vocal fold irregularities and assessment of vocal fold movement/closure patterns, many ENT or voice therapy clinicians will favour using a rigid endoscope with stroboscopy as this produces higher quality imaging and a magnified view of the vocal folds. It does not, however, allow detailed evaluation of vocal tract function during speech and singing.[86]

The purpose of an endoscopy protocol used by a voice therapy clinician is to assess vocal function in relation to speech and, where appropriate, singing. Using a standard protocol for all assessments has merit in that the clinician learns to identify the meaning of and compare particular laryngeal gestures by observing a variety of patterns of phonatory physiology. Many clinicians will have devised their own local protocols and may use slightly different versions depending on the type of voice clinic in which they are working. A shorter protocol will be appropriate when a clear structural or neurogenic cause for the dysphonia is immediately identified. Where the differential diagnosis is less clear or where the primary diagnosis involves a muscle tension dysphonia a more detailed evaluation will be necessary, particularly if therapy techniques are being trialled as part of the protocol.

It is recognized that judgements made during EEL and the resulting evaluations are by their nature subjective. Attempts have been made to develop systems which are more objective[93] but there is no one method commonly used in the clinical setting. It is also the case that patients (particularly those who find the procedures difficult to tolerate) may not produce their habitual vocal tract gestures during the endoscopy. This is especially likely if there is a noticeable change in their vocal quality before and during the examination.

Some of the earliest authors to comment on the advantages of using endoscopy during voice therapy[94] point out the advantages of being able to observe normal and disordered laryngeal physiology.

The first published protocol which addressed and evaluated vocal function in detail was described by Colton and Casper.[7] This included observing the larynx at rest, during deep inspiration, producing sustained vowels, and during a variety of phonatory tasks including pitch change as well as non-phonatory laryngeal behaviour. These were followed by a period of 'diagnostic therapy' during which the patient would be asked to produce voice using various therapy techniques with the aim of eliciting improved vocal function.

Koschkee and Rammage[10] proposed counting and spontaneous speech be included in a standard protocol and Koufman[69] added other vocal tasks, including yawning/sighing/vocal fry/whistling and sniffing as well as reproducing the voice problem as part of the protocol. Some authors[87,95] suggest repeating each vocal manoeuvre several times to assess consistency.

Colton and Estill[96] investigated the vocal manoeuvres of singers using techniques including laryngeal X-rays, voice signal analysis, EMG, electroglottography, and, significantly, fibre-optic EEL. Observed manoeuvres included movements of the lips, tongue, larynx, soft palate, pharynx, laryngeal vestibule, and true vocal folds. This was the first research that documented marked differences in laryngeal gesture for a variety of the vocal qualities that the human voice is able to produce. Creating and using the classification of speech, sob, opera, and twang, Estill found that for the voice to work efficiently, breath, tone, and resonance also had to work together effectively.[97] These observations are strongly supported in the works of other leading voice practitioners.[36,98–100]

Estill's research led to the development of her 'Compulsory Figures', now referred to as 'Figures for Voice Control'. These describe how the vocal tract is configured for various vocal qualities such as speech, falsetto, sob, twang, opera, and belt.[97,101,103] Many voice therapists use the Estill techniques as part of routine clinical practice.

The work of Janice Chapman[36] on 'primal sound' has also been influential in the way clinicians approach the voice. Chapman describes how primal sounds 'emanate from human needs, have emotional triggers, and are part of a whole pattern of responses involving the body and mind in a holistic way'. She explains how when vocalization is associated with primal sound, the adjustments necessary to produce the sound are made automatically. Although this was originally described as an approach for teaching the singing voice, it is also valuable to consider the speaking voice in this way and use these primal sounds to evaluate their effect on the voice.

3.1 University Hospital of South Manchester (UHSM): Endoscopic Evaluation of the Larynx

The Endoscopic Evaluation of the Larynx protocol using a flexible endoscope was developed in order to design a systematic approach to the assessment of vocal function in individuals presenting with dysphonia. It is not specifically designed to be a detailed stroboscopic assessment, as protocols for this are already available and in widespread clinical use.[91,92] The full protocol can be found in Section 3.7.

The protocol combines ideas from leading voice practitioners and researchers, deconstructing the vocal mechanism into a series of specific vocal tract gestures that are used in popular vocal training programmes of recent times. It has been developed and refined over several years during use in daily clinical practice. The concept of the use of 'primal sound' or 'emotional intention' (Section 7) is based on the initial ideas of Janice Chapman.[36] These ideas were subsequently developed by Dane Chalfin, who linked them with the vocal tract gestures seen on endoscopic findings.[102]

The protocol allows observations of habitual or default vocal tract patterns for individuals, also termed 'attractor states' by Jo Estill.[103] Inefficient habitual vocal tract patterns can be modified with therapy and vocal training, establishing new, more vocally efficient habits that will enable an individual to reduce the likelihood of experiencing further vocal problems.[1,8,103,104]

The UHSM protocol for the spoken voice can be divided into eight sections of observation:

- vocal tract at rest;
- abduction and adduction of the vocal folds;
- sustained phonation;
- pitch change;
- phonatory onsets;
- laryngopharyngeal gesture in speech;
- laryngopharyngeal gesture in voice figures/primal sounds; and
- diagnostic therapy.

The directions to the patient are consistent and clinicians are guided as to which aspects of the vocal tract structures should be observed at each particular part of the process. Typically this protocol takes three to six minutes to complete. It is very well tolerated by most patients and the vocal tasks can each be repeated several times. However, some individuals do find the process more difficult and the protocol may need to be shortened under these circumstances. It is often patients with extreme tension in the vocal tract who find flexible laryngeal endoscopy challenging. Repeating the procedure once they have started voice therapy and reduced some of the vocal tract constriction can be of benefit and enable better views to be obtained.

3.2 Observing the larynx at rest, adduction, and abduction

Sections 1 and 2 give an opportunity to evaluate the larynx at rest, during abduction, and during adduction. Symmetry of appearance in the larynx is noted along with any signs of laryngopharyngeal reflux and mucous secretions. When evaluating abduction and adduction of the vocal folds it is important to identify not only if there is a palsy or paresis present but whether the adduction of the vocal folds occurs simultaneously or whether there is 'sluggishness' of movement.

Although this is not a medically diagnostic endoscopy protocol, observation of the general laryngeal appearance is informative. If the patient has been assessed in a general ENT clinic rather than a multidisciplinary voice clinic, experienced voice therapy clinicians performing the endoscopy for therapy planning may identify laryngeal abnormalities which have not been detected at the original ENT examination. These must be brought to the attention of the consultant laryngologist as soon as possible.

3.3 Observing phonation and pitch change

Sections 3 and 4 examine vocal fold closure, mucosal wave vibration, and glottic/supraglottic constriction at a medium, high, and low pitch as well as on a pitch glide. Although many of the instructions can be modelled, it is more reliable to ask patients to use a 'comfortable' pitch for the middle pitch without modelling. Some patients will inevitably try to match the pitch modelled by the clinician, resulting minimally in an atypical pitch and vocal strain at worst.

For good quality voicing, the integrity of the vocal fold vibratory margin is of vital importance.[105] Stroboscopy is used for this section of the protocol to allow for detailed information regarding vibratory asymmetries, structural abnormalities, small masses, submucosal scars, and other conditions that are invisible under normal light.[106] Under stroboscopic light it is possible to assess glottic closure patterns, amplitude of vibration, periodicity, and nonvibrating portions of the vocal fold.[105] Observations can be made of any patterns of constriction also present at this stage.[1]

3.4 Observing onsets

Section 5 allows an endoscopic view of the true and false vocal folds during glottal, breathy, and simultaneous onsets. It is helpful to repeat this section twice or three times if the patient tolerates the procedure well. This enables the clinician to judge consistency of the onset patterns. Some patients will not be able to produce the three types of onset differently. For example those with poor glottic closure may produce all three as breathy onsets.

3.5 Observing laryngopharyngeal gesture

Section 6 is intended to elicit connected speech. It would be appropriate to substitute the chosen instructions, which are based on the sentences used in the CAPE-V auditory-perceptual scheme,[33] with any form of connected speech. For patients who find the endoscopic procedure difficult to tolerate, substituting the sentences with counting from one to ten or twenty is a quicker option which they may find less stressful.

For patients who present with intermittent or variable dysphonia, this section is helpful for asking them to reproduce or 'mimic' the voice problem when it does occur. There is no guarantee that the dysphonia they produce at this point is actually typical of their usual dysphonic voice but many patients have very good insight into whether their attempt is in fact typical. It is interesting to observe that some patients, when asked to reproduce their dysphonia, find themselves unable to do so.

Section 7 uses instructions to elicit sounds such as sigh, cry, sob, whinge, twang, and belt. This yields helpful information in evaluating to what extent patients are able to alter laryngopharyngeal gesture following an auditory stimulus. The presence, absence, and degree of changes in vocal fold thickness, vertical laryngeal excursion, pharyngeal tuning, and cricothyroid tilt can all be observed.

3.6 Diagnostic therapy

Section 8 – the therapy techniques trialled here will be dependent on the earlier findings. Using knowledge of how a particular technique works and what it is meant to achieve, the clinician will choose those methods which may have a positive effect on the way the voice is being produced, changing the habitual laryngeal gesture to one which is more optimal to obtain a improvement in perceived auditory quality. If successful, it is often the case that the patient will also hear the vocal change, which in turn helps with motivation for attending therapy. A list of suggested techniques along with their rationale can be found in Chapter 6.

The evaluation pro forma to be used along with the protocol outlines specifically the key elements to be described for a thorough endoscopic evaluation of vocal function. The descriptions of vocal fold closure patterns in section 3 are based on the original work of Hirano and Bless.[91] Diagrammatic pictures of these can be seen in Figure 3.1.

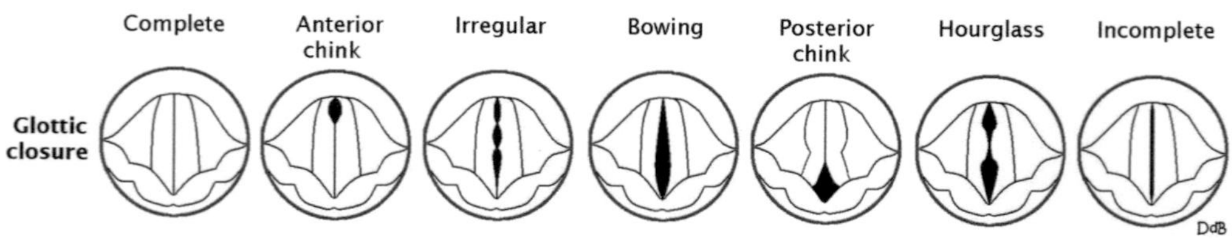

Figure 3.1: Vocal fold closure patterns.

In section 7 of the pro forma, the words in emphasis indicate what would be expected to be observed during the evaluation. This is in accordance with our own extensive clinical observations based on a wide range of clinical voice disorders.

Figure 3.2 shows the expected appearances during endoscopy for each of the manoeuvres in section 7. The dynamic movement which occurs in each of these gestures is captured in a still picture considered typical for each presentation.

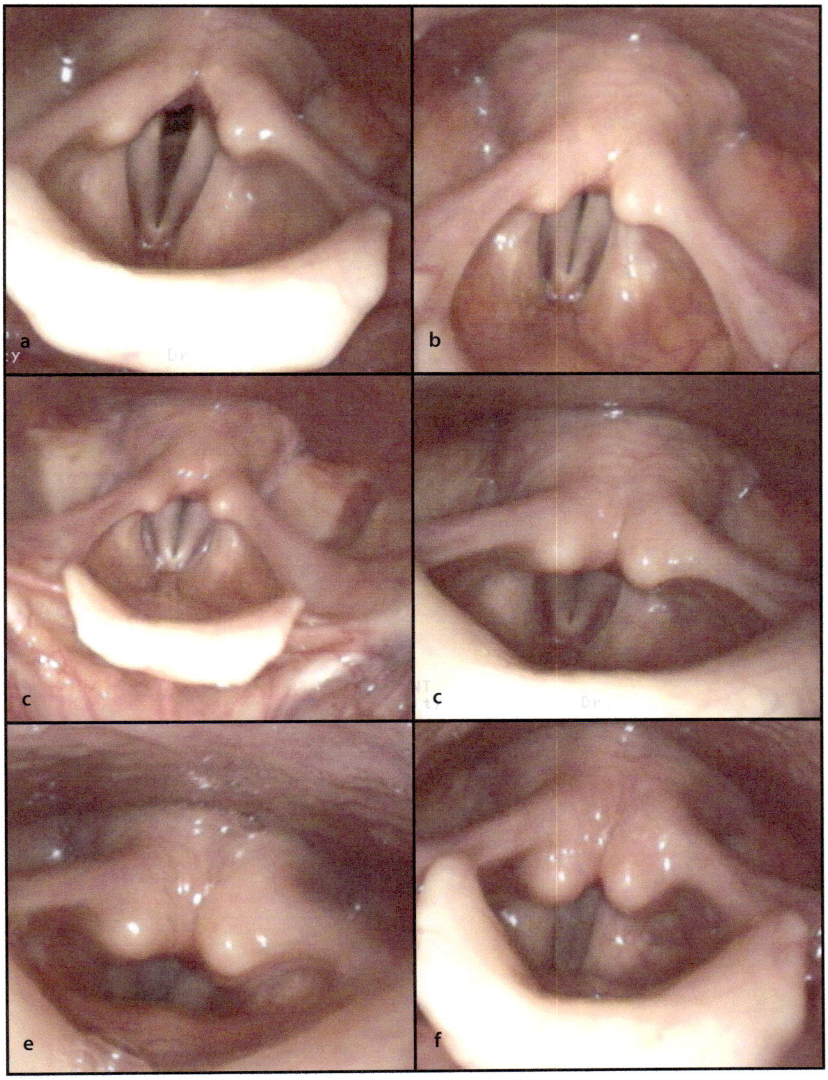

Figure 3.2: Expected appearances during endoscopy. **a.** Sigh. **b.** Whimper (high)/cry. **c.** Whimper (low)/sob. **d.** Whinge/groan. **e.** Twang. **f.** yell/belt.

3.7 UHSM Endoscopic Evaluation of the Larynx protocol

	Direction to Patient	Observations
1.	"Sit comfortably and relax for a moment."	**Observe larynx at rest:** Structural abnormality; vocal fold pathology reflux signs.
2.	"Sniff and sing 'EE' several times as quickly as you can."	**Observe abduction and adduction.**
3a.	"Hold an 'EE' at a comfortable pitch." *(First without stroboscopy, then with.)*	**Observe sustained phonation:** VF closure pattern; mucosal wave; constriction patterns.
3b.	"Do that again on a low pitch." *(Repeat with and without stroboscopy.)*	**Observe sustained phonation (low pitch):** VF closure pattern; mucosal wave; constriction patterns.
3c.	"Do that again on a high pitch." *(Repeat with and without stroboscopy.)*	**Observe sustained phonation (high pitch):** VF closure pattern; mucosal wave; constriction patterns.
4.	"Sing a gentle 'EE' from low to high pitch, and back low again." *(Repeat with and without stroboscopy.)*	**Observe pitch change:** laryngeal excursion; tilt; constriction; tongue backing; pharyngeal muscle-use; pitch breaks.
5a.	"Repeat the following sounds: 'EE EE EE EE EE', 'OO OO OO OO OO'."	**Observe onsets (glottal / hard):** VF and FVF involvement.
5b.	"Repeat the following sounds: 'HEE HEE HEE HEE HEE', 'HOO HOO HOO HOO HOO'."	**Observe onsets (aspirate / breathy):** VF and FVF involvement.
5c.	"Repeat the following sounds: 'YEE YEE YEE YEE YEE', 'YOO YOO YOO YOO YOO'."	**Observe onsets:** simultaneous VF and FVF involvement.

6.	"Repeat these sentences: a. 'The blue spot is on the key again.' b. 'How hard did he hit him?' c. 'We were away a year ago.' d 'We eat eggs every Easter.' e. 'My mama makes lemon muffins.' f. 'Peter will keep at the peak.'" *(If patient's usual dysphonic voice is not produced during the endoscopy procedure ask them to repeat the sentences reproducing the dysphonic voice. Sentences taken from CAPE-V auditory-perceptual analysis.)*	**Observe laryngopharyngeal gesture in speech:** constriction; tongue backing; laryngeal excursion.
7a.	"Sigh from high to low."	**Observe laryngopharyngeal gesture in 'primal' sound (sigh/falsetto):** VF observations; laryngeal gesture observations; pharyngeal observations.
7b.	"Whimper like a tiny puppy."	**Observe laryngopharyngeal gesture in 'primal' sound (high whimper/cry):** VF observations; laryngeal gesture observations; pharyngeal observations.
7c.	"Whimper again and slide down, to a lower pitch."	**Observe laryngopharyngeal gesture in 'primal' sound (low whimper/sob):** VF observations; laryngeal gesture observations; pharyngeal observations.
7d.	"Groan as if you have tummy ache: 'Oh!'"	**Observe laryngopharyngeal gesture in 'primal' sound (whinge/groan):** VF observations; laryngeal gesture observations; pharyngeal observations.

7e.	"Repeat the following sounds: 'Nya Nya Nya Nya Nya' (playground taunt), 'Meeow Meeow Meeow'."	**Observe laryngopharyngeal gesture in 'primal' sound (twang):** VF observations; laryngeal gesture observations; pharyngeal observations.
7f.	"Yell as if someone has just stolen your purse/wallet: 'Eh!'"	**Observe laryngopharyngeal gesture in 'primal' sound (yell/belt):** VF observations; laryngeal gesture observations; pharyngeal observations.
8.	*(Period of diagnostic therapy.)*	**Observe impact/effectiveness of suggested exercises upon laryngopharyngeal gesture/voice.**

3.8 UHSM Endoscopic Evaluation of the Larynx pro forma

Date: ____________________

Patient tolerance of scope:	Excellent	Satisfactory	Poor	
Image quality:	Excellent	Satisfactory	Poor	
Dysphonia severity:	WNL	Mild	Moderate	Severe

WNL - within normal limits *AES - aryepiglottic sphincter* *A-P - anteroposterior* *P-A - posteroanterior*

	Observation	**Evaluation**						
1.	Observe larynx at rest	**Symmetry at rest:**	Vocal folds:	Ventricular folds:	Arytenoids:			
			(0 – symmetric 1 – mild asymmetry 2 – moderate asymmetry 3 – severe asymmetry)					
		Vocal fold pathology:	Yes / No	If yes, describe: ____________				
		Reflux signs:	Mild	Moderate	Severe			
		Mucosal secretions	Normal	Excessive	Dry	Strand(s)		
2.	Abduction/Adduction	**Abduction/Adduction:**	WNL	R palsy / R paresis / R sluggish	L palsy / L paresis / L sluggish			
3a.	Sustained mid-pitch	**VF closure pattern:**	Complete	Ant. chink	Irregular	Post. chink	Hourglass	Incomplete
		Mucosal wave:	Bilateral full	R partial/severe restriction	L partial/severe restriction			
		Constriction:	WNL	Lateral (mild/mod/severe)	A-P (mild/mod/severe)	P-A (mild/mod/severe)		
3b.	Sustained low pitch	**VF closure pattern:**	Complete	Ant. chink	Irregular	Post. chink	Hourglass	Incomplete
		Mucosal wave:	Bilateral full	R partial/severe restriction	L partial/severe restriction			
		Constriction:	WNL	Lateral (mild/mod/severe)	A-P (mild/mod/severe)	P-A (mild/mod/severe)		
3c.	Sustained high pitch	**VF closure pattern:**	Complete	Ant. chink	Irregular	Post. chink	Hourglass	Incomplete
		Mucosal wave:	Bilateral full	R partial/severe restriction	L partial/severe restriction			
		Constriction:	WNL	Lateral (mild/mod/severe)	A-P (mild/mod/severe)	P-A (mild/mod/severe)		

4.	Pitch glide up and down	**Laryngeal vertical excursion:**	Flexible	Static	High-held	Low-held			
		Laryngeal tilt:	WNL	Held vertical	Partial tilt	Held tilted			
		Constriction:	WNL	Lateral (mild/mod/severe)	A-P (mild/mod/severe)	P-A (mild/mod/severe)			
		Tongue backing:	WNL	Mild	Moderate	Severe			
		Pharyngeal wall tuning:	WNL	Absent	Poor	Moderate			
		Pitch breaks:	None	Low range	Mid range	High range			
5a .	Glottal onset	**Vocal folds closure (describe):**							
		False vocal fold closure (describe):							
5b.	Breathy/aspirate onset	**Vocal folds closure (describe):**							
		False vocal fold closure (describe):							
5c.	Simultaneous onset	**Vocal folds closure (describe):**							
		False vocal fold closure (describe):							
6.	Connected speech	**Lateral constriction:**	WNL	Mild	Moderate	Severe			
		A-P/P-A constriction:	WNL	Mild	Moderate	Severe			
		Tongue backing:	WNL	Mild	Moderate	Severe			
		Laryngeal vertical excursion:	Flexible	Static	High-held	Low-held			
7a.	Sigh/falsetto:	VF:	***Stiff***	Thin	Thick			Complete closure of VF:	Yes ***No***
		Larynx:	***Vertical excursion***	Elevated	Lowered	Static	Tilt	Narrow AES	No Tilt
7b.	High whimper/cry:	VF:	Stiff	***Thin***	Thick			Complete closure of VF:	***Yes*** No
		Larynx:	Vertical excursion	***Elevated***	Lowered	Static	***Tilt***	Narrow AES	No Tilt
		Pharynx:	***Narrow***	Normal					
7c.	Low whimper/sob:	VF:	Stiff	***Thin***	Thick			Complete closure of VF:	***Yes*** No
		Larynx:	Vertical excursion	Elevated	***Lowered***	Static	***Tilt***	Narrow AES	No Tilt
		Pharynx:	***Narrow***	Normal					

7d.	Whinge/groan:	VF:	Stiff	Thin	***Thick***			Complete closure of VF:		***Yes***	No
		Larynx:	Vertical excursion		Elevated	Lowered	Static	***Tilt***	Narrow AES	No Tilt	
		Pharynx:	***Narrow***	Normal							
7e.	Twang:	VF:	Stiff	***Thin***	***Thick***			Complete closure of VF:		***Yes***	No
		Larynx:	Vertical excursion		***Elevated***	Lowered	Static	Tilt	***Narrow AES***	No Tilt	
		Pharynx:	Narrow	***Normal***							
7f.	Yell/belt:	VF:	Stiff	Thin	***Thick***			Complete closure of VF:		***Yes***	No
		Larynx:	Vertical excursion		***Elevated***	Lowered	Static	Tilt	***Narrow AES***	No Tilt	
		Pharynx:	***Narrow***	Normal							
8.	Therapy techniques trialled	Impact/ effectiveness of techniques upon laryngopharyngeal gesture / voice quality									

4

Assessment Protocol for the Singing Voice

Sue Jones and Carrie Garrett

Singers are a subset of occupational voice users who are known to be at risk of developing voice disorders[107–109] and who will often present to the voice clinic with problems encompassing both their speaking and singing voice.[110,111]

Other singers present with concerns about their singing voice alone. For vocal professionals dependent on the singing voice for their income this can cause major financial difficulties. There are also many amateur singers for whom singing forms a key element of their quality of life and who can be highly distressed by changes in their voice, which can have a major impact on their social and family life.

The typical concerns of singers presenting with voice problems include:

- loss of pitch and/or dynamic range;
- breathy voice;
- loss of clarity of tone;
- vocal fatigue or reduced vocal stamina;
- discomfort or pain in neck and/or throat;
- change in resonance;
- constricted sound/strain; and
- changes to vibrato.

These can all be symptoms of muscle tension and problems with function of the larynx. However, it is essential to ensure there is no underlying pathology which has resulted in a secondary muscle tension dysphonia rather than muscle tension being the primary cause of the singing problem. Glottic insufficiency is known to give rise to supraglottic hyperfunction as a compensatory manoeuvre.[8] Repetition of ineffective patterns of voicing during particular vocal tasks over a prolonged period of time may cause such problems for singers due to their speaking voice patterns, their singing voice patterns , or a combination.[6,99] As Sataloff[111] states:

> Too frequently, all the expert training in support, muscular control, and projection is not applied to a singer's speaking voice. Unfortunately, the resultant voice strain impacts on the singing as well as the speaking voice.

Underlying structural abnormalities may require surgical intervention. The voice of a singer is likely to be more affected by a small vocal fold lesion than someone who does not have to perform as a vocal athlete. Singers may also be more affected than the average voice user by minor amounts of laryngopharyngeal reflux. Potential laryngeal surgery will be discussed by the patient primarily with the laryngologist, although the voice therapist will be able to offer advice on pre- and post-operative therapy. The voice therapist needs to understand that the potential implications of vocal fold surgery for singers can be significant. Some singers will choose not to go ahead with surgery having considered the likely benefits and possible detriments.

4.1 Problems with pitch

This is one of the most common concerns of singers presenting with vocal difficulties. The ability, or lack thereof, to sing smoothly across the vocal pitch range is of great concern to many singers, particularly those learning their trade and performing in a more amateur capacity. Sometimes referred to by singers as 'switching between vocal qualities', they may describe being able to sing in the lower and upper part of their range but may experience 'cutting out' or a 'dead patch' in the middle of their range. The terms 'chest register' and 'head register' are often used by singers in clinic. The transition between these two registers is referred to as the 'passaggio'. Changes in vocal register are achieved by alterations in the vibratory pattern of the vocal cords. As the register changes there is a 'switch' between 'thick' and 'thin' fold phonation. If this adjustment in vocal fold vibration is not controlled then the voice will be unstable.

The vocal mechanism moves and adjusts to facilitate contact of the true vocal folds across an individual's pitch range. Lack of balance between biomechanics and aerodynamics at different pitches causes 'pitch breaks' and the singer feels as if they have intermittently lost control of their voice. Typically, if a singer is ill-equipped mentally to deal with momentary vocal instability, they may tense up, anticipating further difficulty. This in turn causes glottic instability across register changes and the problem is perpetuated: a vicious circle.

One of the techniques commonly used to remedy problems with pitch is 'sirening'. Estill and McDonald Klimek[97] describe expectation of a healthy, flexible vocal mechanism for the purpose of changing pitch during a siren. There will be observable changes in vocal fold mass, tension, and length. Contraction of the cricothyroid muscle, where the thyroid and cricoid cartilages move closer together, results in the vocal folds becoming elongated and thinned. This facilitates an increased rate of mucosal wave vibration resulting in a higher pitch.[111] This maneouvre is commonly referred to as 'tilt' and is a key aspect of the singing voice. Tilt is often visible during endoscopic evaluation of the larynx, as the arytenoids rise slightly and there is a slightly improved view of the laryngeal vestibule whilst the singer maintains this gesture. In this position, a singer can increase the stiffness of the vocal fold body by contracting the thyroarytenoid muscle. This also serves to shorten the wave cycle and help the singer achieve the higher frequencies.

The optimal position of the larynx during pitch change has been highly debated over the years. Some practitioners feel that the position of the larynx should not vary substantially with pitch changes, and that raising of the larynx with ascending pitch is evidence of technical dysfunction.[105] Estill, however, describes vertical excursion of the larynx as an essential part of pitch change.[103] Clinical observations would indicate that most professional singers have highly flexible larynges, particularly for the more dynamic contemporary vocal styles and musical theatre genre. Further research into variety of flexibility for different vocal musical genres may need to be carried out to answer this question more precisely and in more detail.

Extreme muscular involvement of the tongue, with the tongue pulling backwards when singing, may indicate improper voice use.[105] Changes in resonance to create specific vowel sounds and voice qualities depend on a singer's ability to change the shape of their vocal tract. A combination of larynx, tongue, and soft palate positioning and the use of the pharyngeal constrictor muscles allow a singer to tune formants in their sound (a formant is a concentration of acoustic energy around a particular frequency, each corresponding to a resonance in the vocal tract).[98,99,112] The extent of use of the pharyngeal constrictor muscles is another important component to observe during singing. The most vocally athletic will usually demonstrate the most intense pharyngeal activity. Where singers are struggling with their voice and describe their tone as 'lacking depth' there is often little or no pharyngeal activity.

If an individual has difficulty with control of resonance it is likely there is incorrect use of these structures during voicing, with hyperfunction as a likely outcome. In an effort to compensate for dysfunction at the level of the vocal fold, singers often modify their technique in the neck and the supraglottic vocal tract.[105] A common error is to retract the tongue and tighten the cervical muscles. This only serves to decrease vocal efficiency and increase the risk of vocal strain.

4.2 Singer's protocol

The singer's protocol should be used in addition to the EEL protocol for speech and not on its own. It is essential to explore how a singer uses their speaking voice as this may be making a significant contribution to their singing difficulties. The term 'dyscanto' has been selected in order for the clinician to be able to differentiate the severity of the problems with the sound of the singing voice from those of the speaking voice. The clinician will need to consider whether singers should be seated or standing for this part of the protocol. Karnell[2] recommends that singers should do warm-up exercises to optimize their vocal performance before the endoscopy and suggests that they will perform best if standing during the examination. In clinical practice this may be difficult as the relative heights of the singer and endoscopist need to be taken into consideration in obtaining a good quality image. It can also be problematic to achieve continuously good views of the vocal tract when singers are vocally athletic, particularly those singing pop and rock genres.

Section 9 asks the singer to glide from a low note to a high note and back. This should be repeated several times, encouraging the singer to extend the pitch range at both the lower and upper ends of the scale as far as possible. The purpose of this is to observe the laryngeal gesture during the pitch change. Vertical laryngeal excursion, cricothyroid tilt, unnecessary constriction, excessive tongue backing, pharyngeal constriction, and pitch breaks should all be observed and commented on.

Section 10 instructs the singer to perform what is effectively a messa di voce, but in two sections – singing /i/ on a comfortable pitch and gradually increasing and then decreasing the volume. Breath support must be adjusted to manage the change in intensity required whilst maintaining the consistent pitch. The extent of the change in volume can be described as well as any resultant breaks in phonation and both lateral and antero-posterior constriction. Vibrato can also be monitored during this maneouvre.

Western operatic singers normally perform messa di voce using one of two different vocal techniques. In the first approach, the vocal folds are brought to their optimum state and are kept there for the entire exercise. The sound quality remains constant throughout the phonation without breathy initiation. The second technique involves a breathy beginning followed by a gradual closing of the vocal folds during crescendo and a gradual opening of the folds during decrescendo. The breathy sound eventually attains full timbre.[113]

Section 11 asks the singer to perform two pieces from their repertoire – one which they feel relatively comfortable with and one which showcases their singing difficulties. A verse and chorus of each song is usually sufficient. Performers who have lost their confidence as a result of their vocal problems can be reluctant to sing and need to be reassured that their voice is not being judged but that being able to observe the vocal gestures they are using during singing will enable a more thorough evaluation of the problem for planning vocal rehabilitation. This is the opportunity to observe directly what happens in the vocal tract when the singer encounters their specific difficulty.

Section 12 acts as an opportunity to trial therapy techniques during singing. This will be dependent on what has been seen during both the speaking and singing protocol and the clinician choosing the appropriate techniques to alleviate the difficulty. For example, a common difficulty experienced by singers who are unable to reach the higher part of their range is a lack of laryngeal vertical excursion and limited cricothyroid tilt. Asking them to repeat the song using the 'cry' technique[97] may produce a more effective laryngeal gesture and better sound. Kayes refers to this as a permutation of sob quality, adopting a higher laryngeal position.[114]

4.3 Vocal genres

The work of Estill[97] and Sadolin[115] has shown that the singing voice can be produced in a wide variety of genres and the voice can remain healthy. Different vocal styles require diverse use of the vocal apparatus. For example, observations of the vocal tract during singing clearly show that the laryngeal position for 'belt' is not the same as that for opera. Voice therapists are likely to come across performers from a range of musical backgrounds including classical, musical theatre, pop, rock, and band singers. Each of these will have their own particular needs and approaches to their work.[112] However, singers in today's commercial environment can be asked to sing a variety of styles even within one performance and this requirement for crossover in vocal styles can lead to problems, especially for those who lack training. Research into the use of distortion effects in singing, traditionally thought to have been damaging to the voice, have shown that this is not necessarily the case and distortions such as 'growl' can be produced healthily providing the singer is taught to do this safely.[115,116]

Koufman[117] found that the degree of muscle tension used by singers in various genres was highly variable, with the least muscle tension being employed in choral music and the most muscle tension seen in rock and gospel music. This research also found that singers who had undergone formal training were likely to have significantly lower muscle tension than those who had not undergone training.

It is therefore essential for the voice therapist working with the vocal rehabilitation of singers to have a good understanding of the types of vocal styles used by an individual and how these will be produced differently by the vocal tract. Some vocal styles will require what appears to be undesirable constriction in the laryngopharynx. However, this apparent constriction may be a necessary part of the gesture required to achieve the desired vocal quality. Providing this constriction can be released easily by the singer it is not a problem. It only becomes an issue when the constriction is present all the time and begins to affect other aspects of performance, and potentially the speaking voice as well. Figure 4.1 shows distortion in singing in a healthy larynx followed immediately by release of the distortion into an open laryngeal gesture.

Another client group seen in the voice clinic setting are the 14–19 year old students who are keen to pursue a musical career, be that in the classical, musical theatre, or popular music environment. These students, who are just developing their voices, come to the clinic usually because they are experiencing problems with vocal tone and/or vocal stamina. Sometimes they are sent after they have attended auditions for music courses and the tutors auditioning them have expressed concern there may be an underlying vocal pathology. After taking the appropriate information and a thorough endoscopic examination of the larynx, the voice therapy clinician will decide whether vocal rehabilitation is required, but in all cases the student should be advised to seek coaching from a singing teacher familiar with the singing style they wish to adopt.

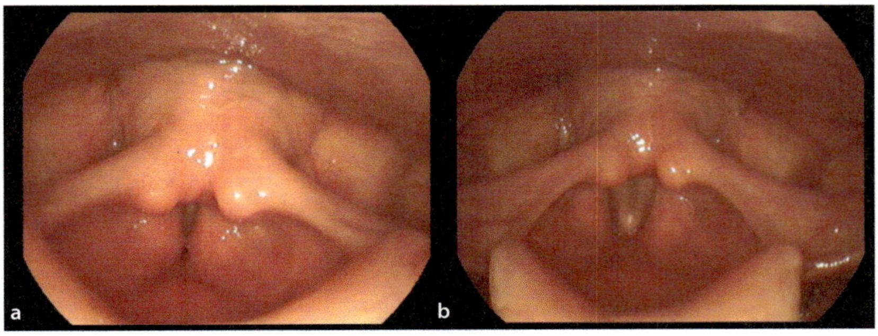

Figure 4.1: a. distortion in singing. **b.** release of constriction.

4.4 UHSM Endoscopic Evaluation of the Larynx for Singers – additional protocol

	Direction to Patient	Observations
9.	"Sing a gentle 'EE' from the lowest note you can make to the highest note you can make, and back low again." *(Repeat several times encouraging a greater pitch range each time.)*	**Observe pitch change:** laryngeal excursion; tilt; constriction; tongue backing; pharyngeal muscle use; pitch breaks.
10a.	"Sing an 'EE' at a comfortable pitch and become louder whilst holding the note."	**Observe volume change:** volume change; phonation breaks; constriction; vibrato.
10b.	"Sing an 'EE' at a comfortable pitch and become quieter whilst holding the note."	**Observe volume change:** volume change; phonation breaks; constriction; vibrato.
11a.	"Sing a verse and chorus of a piece you feel comfortable singing at the moment."	**Observe flexibility of laryngopharyngeal gesture and over-all coordination whilst singing.**
11b.	"Sing a verse and chorus of a piece that is causing you problems at the moment."	**Observe flexibility of laryngopharyngeal gesture and over-all coordination whilst singing.**
12.	*(Period of diagnostic therapy to facilitate improved laryngopharyngeal gesture for singing.)*	**Observe impact/effectiveness of suggested exercises upon laryngopharyngeal gesture/voice.**

4.5 UHSM Endoscopic Evaluation of the Larynx for Singers – additional pro forma

Patient Details	Date: ____________				
	Patient tolerance of scope:	Excellent		Satisfactory	Poor
	Dyscanto severity:	WNL	Mild	Moderate	Severe

	Observation	Evaluation				
9.	Pitch range	**Laryngeal excursion:**				
		Tilt:				
		Constriction:				
		Tongue backing:				
		Pharyngeal wall tuning:				
		Pitch breaks:				
10a.	'EE' increasing in loudness	**Change in volume:**	None	Partial	Full	
		Phonation breaks:	Yes	No	Comments: ____________	
		Constriction:	WNL	Lateral (mild/mod/severe)		A-P/P-A (mild/mod/severe)
		Vibrato:	Natural	Excessive	None	
10b.	'EE' decreasing in loudness	**Change in volume:**	None	Partial	Full	
		Phonation breaks:	Yes	No	Comments: ____________	
		Constriction:	WNL	Lateral (mild/mod/severe)		A-P/P-A (mild/mod/severe)
		Vibrato:	Natural	Excessive	None	
11a.	Song excerpt (comfortable)	**Comments:**				
11b.	Song excerpt (problematic)	**Comments:**				
12.	Period of diagnostic therapy	**Comments:**				

5

Muscle Tension Dysphonia

The term 'muscle tension dysphonia' (MTD) is now widely in use and is the term preferred here. It is, however, a very broad definition and encompasses a wide range of potential presentations. MTD may be primary or secondary in origin and it is sometimes difficult to differentiate between the two in clinical practice. Supraglottic hyperfunction seen during endoscopic evaluation of the larynx must be carefully evaluated to ensure there is no underlying problem at the glottic level.[118] An accurate picture of an MTD results from a thorough case history, general observations, a detailed auditory-perceptual analysis, appropriate instrumental analysis, and excellent laryngeal imaging. The therapist will need to set aims and objectives for voice therapy with the patient using the information obtained from all of the above.

In 2006 the American Speech–Language–Hearing Association (ASHA) published the *Classification Manual for Voice Disorders*.[119] This volume provides a systematic overview and classification of over 120 conditions affecting the voice. These are summarised by Stemple, Glaze, and Klaben[95] into eight major groups:

1. structural pathologies;
2. inflammatory conditions;
3. trauma and injury;
4. systemic conditions;
5. aerodigestive conditions;
6. psychiatric and psychological conditions;
7. neurological conditions; and
8. 'other disorders of voice'.

This final group includes vocal misuse, vocal fatigue, ventricular phonation, paradoxical vocal fold motion, and MTD, both primary and secondary.

Other authors[1,87] have emphasised the muscle tension aspects of dysphonia and adopted the 'musculo-skeletal' approach in which voice disorders are seen as being caused by misuse or poor coordination of the muscles involved in respiration, phonation, resonance, and articulation.

Morrison and Rammage classified 'muscle misuse' voice disorders into six main types.[120] These are described as:

1. laryngeal isometric disorder – generalised tension in the laryngeal muscles often associated with a posterior glottic chink (see Figure 5.1a);
2. (a) lateral glottic contraction – hyperadduction of the vocal folds associated with vocal fatigue (see Figure 5.1b), and (b) lateral supraglottic contraction – similar to Type 2a but with adduction of the false vocal folds (see Figure 5.1c);
3. antero-posterior supraglottic contraction – can vary in degree and is associated with effortful voice lacking vocal stamina (see Figure 5.1d);
4. conversion aphonia/dysphonia – vocal folds are held in a partially adducted position on phonation but do not meet (see Figure 5.1e);
5. psychogenic dysphonia with bowed vocal folds – bowing is not due to presbyphonia and normal phonation can be achieved with therapy techniques (see Figure 5.1f); and
6. adolescent transitional dysphonia – high, tense larynx with inappropriately high pitch (see Figure 5.1g).

More recently Koufman[69] has suggested four types of laryngeal muscle tension patterns (MTP).

MTP I is characterized by a gap between the vocal folds during phonation with a potentially larger gap in the posterior third of the glottis. This is similar to the laryngeal isometric disorder described by Morrison and Rammage, who refer to an 'open glottic chink'. Koufman suggests that this pattern can be observed in patients with vocal fold nodules and in some patients with conversion aphonia.

MTP II is described as approximation of the false vocal folds to varying degrees. This can range from mild constriction of the false vocal folds with the true vocal folds still visible to, at the other extreme, severe false vocal fold constriction where they may actually vibrate – a condition sometimes referred to as

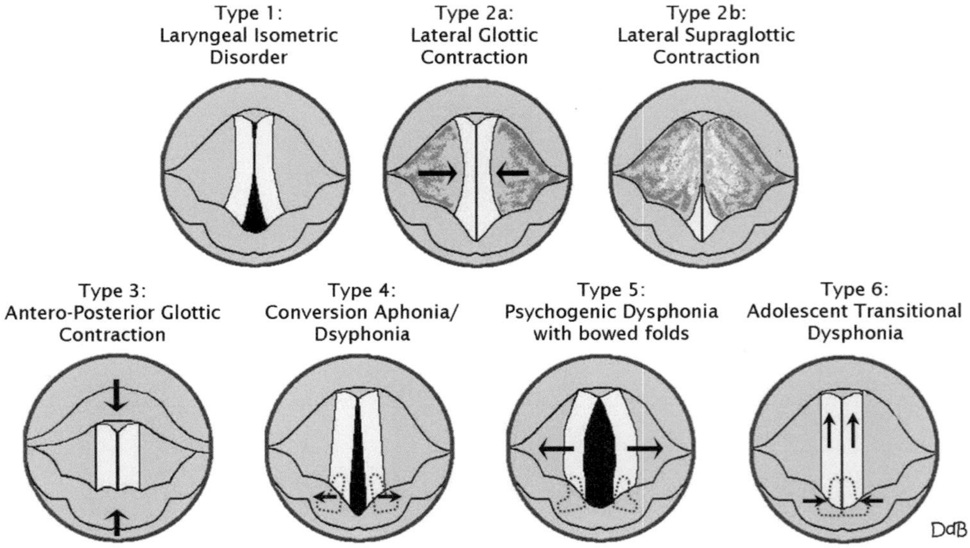

Figure 5.1: Morrison and Rammage Muscle Tension Patterns

'dysphonia plicae ventricularis'. Koufman suggests that MTP II is a compensatory action for glottal incompetence, especially in its more severe form.

MTP III is characterized by antero-posterior constriction of the supraglottic area, with the arytenoids drawn forward towards the epiglottic petiole but with the vocal folds still visible to some extent. This is similar to Type 3 in Morrison and Rammage's classification system.

MTP IV is seen where the arytenoids are brought forward onto the epiglottic petiole and there is no view of the vocal folds. Koufman suggests that this is the least common but often the most severe of the MTPs.

Figure 5.2 illustrates these four types of muscle tension pattern.

McGlashan et al.[121] put forward an alternative way of considering the aetiology of voice disorders and the interaction between the various causal elements, aiming to determine which are primary causes of an individual's dysphonia and what are the potential secondary effects. For example, a primary muscle tension imbalance involving hard glottal attack and/or a posterior glottic chink may lead to the development of a structural abnormality such as vocal fold nodules or polyps. Alternatively, chronic inflammation of the vocal folds may lead to a muscle tension imbalance as the patient develops compensatory supraglottic constriction in an attempt to produce clearer vocal quality.

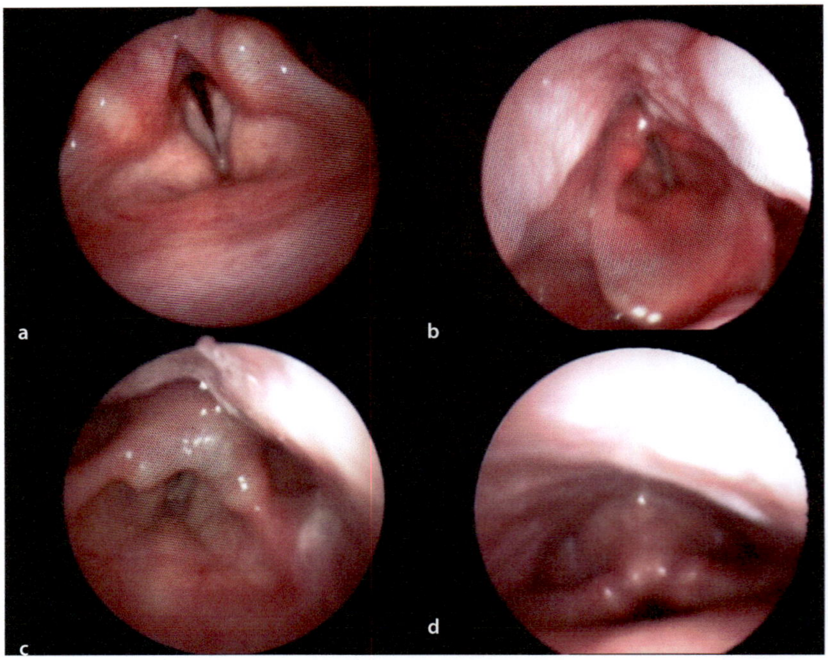

Figure 5.2: Muscle tension patterns. **a.** MTP I. **b.** MTP II. **c.** MTP III. **d.** MTP IV.

Whilst the classification systems referred to above are a useful starting point, patients do not always present with phonatory muscle patterns which easily fit into categories and it is therefore helpful to adopt a descriptive system in order to plan therapy as suggested in the protocols in Chapter 3 and Chapter 4. What is commonly described as antero-posterior (AP) constriction may be more accurately described as postero-anterior (PA) constriction and it is for this reason both these terms are used in the evaluation pro forma (Chapter 3). PA constriction, where the arytenoids move towards the epiglottic petiole, is extremely common in MTP and can mask glottal insufficiency. True AP constriction occurs when the arytenoids are maintained upright and the epiglottic petiole appears to move posteriorly covering the anterior portion of the vocal folds whilst the posterior part of the glottis including the vocal processes remain visible. Some patients may present with both AP and PA constriction, so only the mid third of the vocal folds are visible (Sara Harris – personal communication).

5.1 Primary muscle tension dysphonia

Typically a primary MTD will have no underlying vocal fold pathology and is caused by vocal tract muscle misuse patterns. This leads to an inefficient habitual state of voicing, which in turn leads to dysphonia. These voicing patterns can be affected by muscle tension not only in the larynx but in the whole body; hence it is essential to assess the contributory elements of posture, breathing, phonation, resonance, pitch, loudness, and articulation.[34] Many of the patients referred to voice therapists will come with a diagnosis of 'normal larynx'. This usually means the examiner did not find any structural, neuromuscular, or inflammatory abnormalities during the laryngeal examination. However, the patient remains dysphonic and a cause for the dysphonia needs to be determined. It is useful for the voice therapist to know exactly how the voice is being produced and what patterns of muscle tension may be present.

Primary MTD usually responds well to a combination of indirect and direct therapy techniques and these are described in detail in Chapter 6.

5.2 Secondary muscle tension dysphonia

A secondary MTD occurs where there is recruitment of supralaryngeal muscles owing to an underlying problem at vocal fold level. Glottal insufficiency (an inability to close the vocal folds) may occur for a wide variety of reasons, including inflammatory changes such as laryngopharyngeal reflux, chronic laryngitis, or Reinke's oedema; neuromuscular conditions such as a palsy or paresis; or structural changes in the form of vocal fold lesions. The supraglottic structures are then recruited in an attempt to attain vocal fold closure. Where it is not possible to view the vocal folds because of excess supraglottic constriction, techniques to release the constriction may help to obtain a better image during endoscopy. A view of the vocal folds is essential in order to exclude any underlying glottal insufficiency.

In cases of secondary MTD management will be made jointly by the voice clinic team and the patient. Voice therapy may be very limited in its efficacy until the underlying lesion or glottal insufficiency is resolved. If surgery is the treatment of choice, pre-operative voice therapy may be of help in reducing the compensatory vocal tract gestures followed by post-operative therapy to ensure use of the best vocal quality with minimum effort.

Koufman employed the term 'unloading' to refer to reducing this type of compensatory laryngeal behaviour during endoscopy in order to make a more accurate diagnostic assessment.[122] A number of techniques, described below, can be effective in achieving this aim. Not all methods will be effective with all patients depending on how comfortable they are during the examination, the severity of their dysphonia, and how easy it is for them to alter their vocal tract habitual state.

The techniques to reduce compensatory laryngeal muscle tension patterns include:

- Inhalation/exhalation: the clinician instructs the patient to breathe in and out whilst voicing. The vocal fold mucosa is thrown upwards on inspiration and this will often reveal any lesion on the undersurface of the vocal folds.
- Yawn: the clinician asks the patient to 'yawn gently' without voicing. This technique lowers the larynx and often releases false vocal fold constriction, enabling a better view of the vocal folds.
- Giggle/laugh: the patient is asked to 'giggle or snigger silently' to release false vocal fold constriction.
- In-breath of delight: the patient is asked to take a breath quickly as if surprised. This can also release supraglottic constriction.
- Silent inspiration: the patient is asked to breathe deeply but quietly and to 'open the throat' if possible. This lowers the larynx and, again, reduces supraglottic constriction.
- Laughter: the best way to reduce supralaryngeal constriction is if the patient laughs naturally during the endoscopic procedure. This cannot be forced, but spending time preparing the patient for the examination and establishing a good relationship can encourage it to occur.

5.3 Emotion and the voice

It is widely acknowledged amongst voice clinicians that emotion may play a role in the aetiology and maintenance of dysphonia. It is recognized that in some instances the primary cause of the voice disorder can be related to a psychological or psychiatric condition, and some authors have described methods of assessment and specific voice therapy management in these cases.[123,124] Even where the primary aetiology of the dysphonia is not psychogenic, stress and anxiety can play a role in exacerbating symptoms and many patients will state that their voice is worse when they feel anxious.

Voice clinicians should always take into account the role emotions may play in an individual's voice disorder. Stress and anxiety can lead to excess tension in the body generally, which may manifest itself in the extrinsic and intrinsic laryngeal muscles contributing to the dysphonic symptoms. This in turn may be observed as part of the endoscopic examination.

5.4 Summary

Muscle tension dysphonia may be primary or secondary, and the factors contributing to an individual's voice problem may well be multifactorial. The voice therapist must be aware of all potential contributing factors but also make sure each is considered carefully in terms of the extent of its effect on the voice. Jumping to conclusions before reflecting on all available information should be avoided as this can lead to key elements being missed, inaccurate voice therapy diagnosis, and inappropriate treatment. This is especially important when a patient presents with intermittent or episodic dysphonia. If a patient presents with a normal voice at their clinic appointment and the endoscopic evaluation of the larynx on the day shows normal structure and function, it may be prudent to re-examine them when they do present with the dysphonia in order to complete a thorough assessment.

Figure 5.3 illustrates how the interaction of various factors should be considered when making a differential diagnosis of muscle tension dysphonia.

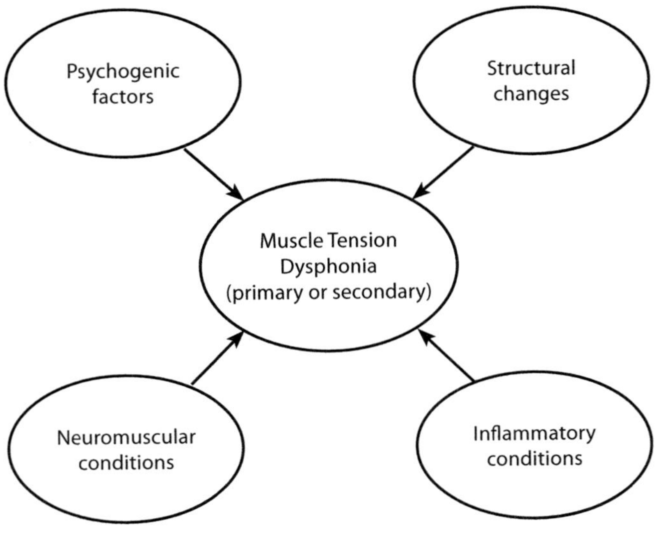

Figure 5.3: Muscle tension dysphonia.

6

Voice Therapy Techniques

6.1 Principles of voice therapy

One of the earliest books dedicated exclusively to voice disorders, written by Albert T. Murphy in 1964,[125] describes how prior to the 1930s the art of voice therapy was initially practised by a small group of laryngologists, singing teachers, drama teachers, and elocutionists all with a particular interest in 'vocal defects'. Therapy techniques relied largely on modelling together with the use of drills and exercises. Interestingly, Murphy lists 40 therapy techniques. Boone later described 24 voice therapy techniques which included both indirect and direct methods.[126] Many of these are similar to those described by Murphy, but there is more detail on the application to specific voice disorders.

Recently there has been a plethora of research into voice production and vocal rehabilitation which has provided us with the scientific underpinning behind familiar vocal therapy techniques. However, most of our treatment techniques continue to have their origins in the past.

Stemple, Glaze, and Klaben[127] outline the following four approaches to voice therapy.

1. symptomatic: therapy techniques are chosen to modify signs and symptoms of the dysphonia which have been observed during the assessment;
2. psychogenic: therapy focuses on identifying and modifying the psychosocial factors associated with the onset and continuation of the voice problem;
3. hygienic: therapy is based on identifying the etiologic factors for the dysphonia and working to eliminate them; and

4. physiologic: the use of direct voice therapies which are used to modify physiological gestures of the vocal mechanism.

Clinicians will most often employ several, if not all, of these approaches during a course of voice therapy and Stemple refers to this as the 'eclectic' approach.

6.2 Therapy techniques

Many authors have written about voice therapy techniques, outlining general principles, methods, and applications.[6,8,34,95,104,128–131] Other clinicians and researchers have described their own specific approaches such as the Accent Method,[132] Figures for Voice Control,[97,103] Voicecraft,[134] Resonant Voice Therapy,[135] Vocal Function Exercises,[95] and the Lee Silverman approach.[136]

Indirect voice therapy techniques are well described and include those which encompass education and explanation, vocal care awareness and advice, elimination of adverse vocal behaviours, auditory training, general relaxation, and counselling. All these factors are important to take into account in an overall therapy management plan and some patients will benefit from more of an indirect approach than others.

Direct therapy techniques comprise those which result in an alteration of the positioning of the structures of the vocal tract and of co-ordination of breathing and phonation. Use of these techniques can change the way the voice is being produced, leading to improved vocal quality. Before voice therapists used endoscopic evaluation of the larynx the effects of these direct techniques on the voice was judged by auditory-perceptual analysis alone. Under endoscopic examination the change in laryngeal gestures can also be observed. Dejonckere[137] refers to 'vocal plasticity' as a method where vocal parameters are changed during the vocal assessment in order to test which are the most effective in obtaining rapid improvement in voice quality. These are then used as a basis for therapy management. He describes perceptual assessment as the main method of evaluation, however using endoscopic findings in additional to perceptual analysis can make a major contribution to this process

It is widely accepted that voice therapy is effective in the management of dysphonia. In studies on the efficacy of voice therapy Carding found that although both indirect and direct therapy techniques were of value; the most significant improvement was shown where both indirect and direct therapy techniques were used.[138,139] In 2013 Gartner-Schmidt[140] reported that in clinical practice where voice therapists were free to choose the component parts of voice therapy for individual patients, they adopted direct treatment techniques for more than 75 percent of the time. Rattenbury et al[63] demonstrated that voice therapy using transnasal flexible laryngoscopy was both effective and more efficient than traditional voice therapy in terms of the amount of time required to achieve a positive outcome.

The purpose of the EEL protocol is to provide a systematic description of vocal function during speech and singing, in order to inform the clinician about which therapy techniques are most likely to successfully modify the inefficient laryngopharyngeal gestures and substitute them with more efficient ones. The effect of this process should be improved vocal quality and stamina as well as a reduction in vocal tract discomfort. From observations made during the first seven sections of the protocol the voice therapy clinician will form a hypothesis as to the component factors contributing to the dysphonia.

Completing the protocol itself is likely to provide a great deal of information about the effectiveness of various therapy techniques as a range of vocal fold onset patterns as well as primal sound stimuli are used. A change in vocal tract gesture and vocal quality may already have been observed. The voice therapist may wish to repeat and/or extend some of these techniques during the diagnostic therapy section, and will also use other approaches which result in adjustments to the vocal gestures. For example, if the EEL shows evidence of the voice being produced with excess glottal attack and constriction of the false vocal folds, therapy techniques to reduce laryngeal and supralaryngeal constriction can be trialled.

Various authors have suggested techniques which could be used during the diagnostic therapy section of the EEL protocol.[6,69,87] Listed below are some of the most useful therapy techniques, together with references, to trial during the period of diagnostic therapy in the EEL protocol along with which changes in the vocal tract gesture would be expected. It is important to note that not all patients do produce these changes and this can be informative in itself. Many voice therapy techniques have multiple effects and do not just change one feature viewed during endoscopy. Some techniques can be used for apparently opposite purposes and still have a positive effect. There are also many techniques which achieve the same overall aim and some patients respond better to some methods than others.

6.2.1 Techniques which improve vocal fold closure/establish modal voice

- Glottal onset.[103]
- Accent method.[132,141]
- Glottal fry/creak.[104]
- Humming.[95,104,128,135]
- Simultaneous onset.[103]
- Sob/cry.[97]
- Plosive consonant closure.[6]
- Vocal function exercise.[127]
- Twang.[97]

6.2.2 Techniques which reduce glottic and/or false fold constriction

- Silent inspiration.[142]
- Silent giggle/laughter.[103]
- Accent method.[132,141]
- Breath before tone.[103]
- Humming.[95,104,128,135]
- Sob/cry.[97]
- Simultaneous onset.[103]

6.2.3 Techniques which reduce antero-posterior constriction

- Sob.[97]
- Accent method.[132,141]
- Laryngeal manipulation.[35,37,38,39]
- Yawn/sigh.[104]

6.2.4 Techniques which reduce pharyngeal constriction/lower larynx

- Yawn/sigh.[104,143]
- Chewing.[104]
- Sob.[97]
- Laryngeal manipulation.[35,37,38,39]
- Accent method.[132,141]
- Semi-occluded vocal tract exercises.[144]

6.2.5 Techniques which increase cricothyroid tilt

- Sirening.[103]

6.2.6 Techniques which improve voice projection

- Humming.[95,104,128,135]
- Twang.[97]
- Resonance work.[34,135]

Table 6.1 summarises the techniques and the changes expected on endoscopy.

None of these lists are exhaustive and not all techniques will stimulate the same response in each individual. A thorough knowledge of a wide range of techniques and their potential effects will help the clinician to choose effective techniques appropriately. However, for some patients there will be no change in either laryngeal gesture or vocal quality during the endoscopic evaluation. This does not mean voice therapy will be ineffective. Equally, there are some direct therapy techniques that are difficult to trial when the endoscope is in place, particularly those which involve changes in nasality, breathing, or postural patterns.

Endoscopic evaluation of the larynx can also be a very useful biofeedback tool in voice therapy. Maryn et al in 2006[61] conducted a systematic literature review of the effects of biofeedback in voice disorders. The review looked at the effects of acoustic and electromyographic feedback as well as laryngoscopic. They concluded that, although many of the studies had limitations, there was evidence that in general biofeedback methods improved the results of voice therapy. The studies that specifically looked at laryngoscopy as a biofeedback tool all showed it to successfully improve vocal quality and function.[59–62]

In clinical practice it is easy to set up a second monitor linked to the main equipment with a splitter mechanism so that the patient can visualize their vocal tract during the examination should they feel comfortable with this. They are then able to observe the changes in laryngopharyngeal gestures that they make and link these with the auditory changes they hear. This is often very helpful in enabling patients to understand why particular therapy techniques are being used, increasing the motivation for participating in treatment. Individuals who do not wish to view their larynx during the examination may benefit from reviewing the examination on screen with the voice therapist once it the examination finished. This enables the patient and clinician to discuss the findings and allows the patient to gain a better understanding of their dysphonia. However, some patients will decline viewing their own larynx as they find the idea distressing.

	Reduce pharyngeal constriction/lower larynx	Reduce glottic/false vocal fold constriction	Reduce antero-posterior or postero-anterior constriction	Improve vocal fold closure/ establish modal voice	Improve cricothyroid tilt	Improve vocal projection
Silent inspiration		✓				
Silent giggle/laugh		✓				
Yawn/sigh	✓		✓			
Accent method	✓	✓	✓	✓		
Breath before tone		✓				
Plosive consonant closure				✓		
Glottal onset				✓		
Simultaneous onset		✓		✓		
Humming		✓		✓		
Glottal fry/creak				✓		
Sob/whine	✓	✓	✓	✓		
Chewing	✓					
Vocal function exercises				✓		
Laryngeal manuipulation	✓		✓			
Twang				✓		✓
Siren					✓	
Semi-occluded vocal tract exercises	✓					
Resonance work						✓

Table 6.1: Vocal techniques and changes expected upon endoscopy.

7

Endoscopic Evaluation of the Larynx Case Presentations

The following case presentations demonstrate how voice therapy techniques can be used during endoscopic evaluation of the larynx in order to guide voice therapy. In each case the findings were shown to and discussed with the patient following the examination. The visual feedback enabled the patient to understand the purpose of the techniques and motivated him or her to attend for therapy. The figures shown are illustrative of the vocal gestures produced by each patient during the examinations and demonstrate the changes which were elicited by trialling therapy techniques in order to change the laryngeal gesture.

Case 1

Florence, aged 50, worked as a music teacher with primary school children in a British Forces Centre abroad. Following a viral infection she had lost power in her voice and had become unable to sing. A local ENT examination had found an essentially normal larynx with possible bowing of the right vocal cord. She had spent a few weeks initially resting her voice and then had continued working, but with reduced voice use. Florence's voice had recovered to the extent that she was able to return to the classroom and speak quietly but after even a short period of teaching her voice would become inaudible. At the time of attending the voice clinic she was able to teach for only two hours per day and needed amplification at all times. She was extremely concerned about her voice and worried about her future career.

At assessment Florence presented with a breathy, weak, high pitched vocal quality. Her GRBAS score was G3 R0 B2 A2 S2. The vocal folds were consistently held in a 'thin fold' stretched position during all vocal tasks (see Figure 7.1a). On phonation there was a restricted mucosal wave in both vocal folds and incomplete vocal fold closure. Palpation of the neck indicated that the larynx was held high with notable tension in the thyrohyoid and cricothyroid muscles. Her pitch was high and monotone and she was unable to project her voice.

Therapy techniques were trialled with the aim of releasing tension in the vocal folds and lowering the larynx. Yawn/sigh was successful in lowering the larynx and humming reduced vocal fold tension, enabling the vocal folds to vibrate with an increased mass. This enabled Florence to produce a clearer vocal tone with reduced breathiness at a normal pitch during the examination (see Figure 7.1b).

Case 2

Mary, aged 43, was initially referred for speech therapy three months after a possible but unconfirmed cerebro-vascular accident (CVA). At this time she had reported 'struggling to get words out' when stressed. By the time she attended for speech therapy her word-finding difficulties had fully resolved but she had developed a severe dysphonia, which was her main concern. She therefore attended the voice clinic.

At her voice clinic appointment Mary stated that she felt her voice had deteriorated around the time she was admitted to hospital with a possible CVA. She felt that her voice was very variable, ranging from normal to severely dysphonic, but was not aware of any particular pattern to the change. Her GRBAS score was G3 R1 B2 A0 S0. She also had a moderately low pitch and mildly low

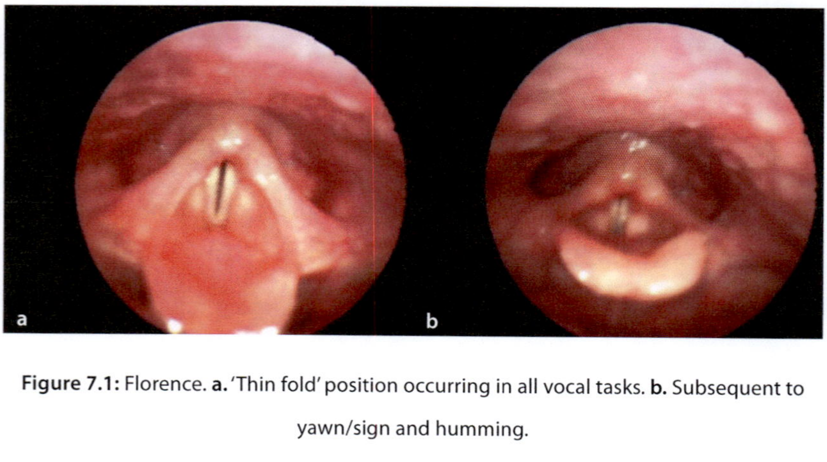

Figure 7.1: Florence. **a.** 'Thin fold' position occurring in all vocal tasks. **b.** Subsequent to yawn/sign and humming.

volume. Mary lived alone and did not use her voice extensively. She had been a heavy smoker but had recently given up. She was on extensive medications including for laryngopharyngeal reflux.

Endoscopic evaluation of the larynx showed a lowered larynx with severe antero-posterior constriction (see Figure 7.2a). At times the vocal folds were obscured entirely but views were obtained demonstrating full vocal fold closure and a full bilateral mucosal wave. Therapy techniques including sob, simultaneous onset, humming, and accent method were trialled. Mary was able to partially release the supraglottic constriction during the procedure and these techniques were then used in her voice therapy sessions (see Figure 7.2b).

Case 3

Peter, aged 36, was a research scientist and lecturer. His work involved giving presentations and chairing meetings. He also had three children under the age of five with whom he used his voice a great deal. Four months before attending the voice clinic he had become severely dysphonic for two months, but had continued to struggle to work. Peter reported that he had experienced similar problems with his voice in the past and described his voice as generally 'weak'. Although his voice had improved in the intervening two months, his vocal stamina was very poor and his voice would deteriorate quickly with use. He described himself as 'straining' to produce his voice most of the time. On the GRBAS scale his voice was rated as G2 R1 B1 A1 S1. His voice was quiet and he found it difficult to project and produce a louder volume.

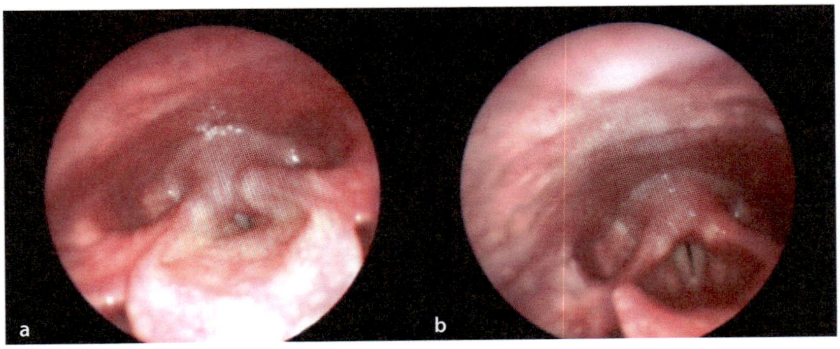

Figure 7.2: Mary. **a.** Lowered larynx with antero-posterior constriction. **b.** Partially released supraglottic constriction.

Peter had been asthmatic since childhood and took asthma medication regularly. He had given up smoking five years previously and described his alcohol intake as moderate.

Endoscopic evaluation of the larynx showed full abduction and adduction of the vocal folds but with some asymmetry of movement of the arytenoid cartilages. There was severe antero-posterior constriction present at all times together with moderate lateral constriction of the vocal folds (see Figure 7.3a). It was difficult to view the vocal folds but unloading techniques (see Chapter 5) allowed enough of a view to establish there was a full bilateral mucosal wave and he could achieve full vocal fold closure. Therapy techniques were trialled aiming to release the severe supraglottic constriction seen during the examination. These included yawn/sigh, humming, sob, and accent method. The changes achieved were very subtle but there was some slight release of antero-posterior constriction, allowing a better view of the length of the vocal folds and an improved laryngeal gesture (see Figure 7.3b).

Case 4

Kathleen, aged 55, had experienced recurrent episodes of dysphonia over a period of several years. She had previously attended the voice clinic service and been diagnosed with intermittent muscle tension dysphonia but had chosen not to have any intervention at that time. She re-presented two years later with worsening dysphonia. At this time her voice was analysed on the GRBAS scale as G2 R2 B1 A0 S1. Her Voice Handicap Index-10 score was 20/40. Kathleen's voice problems were causing difficulty in her work as a receptionist, especially

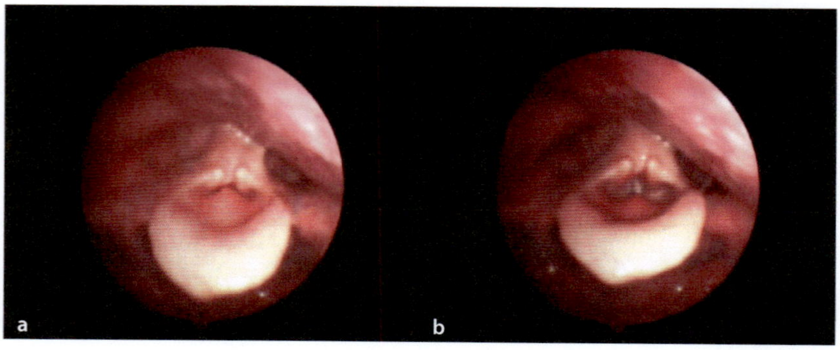

Figure 7.3: Peter. **a.** Antero-posterior constriction with moderate lateral constriction. **b.** Release of antero-posterior constriction.

when she had to use the telephone. Her voice would deteriorate by the end of the day and she found it effortful to speak. She had recently been diagnosed with depression, although she stated this was not entirely due to her voice problems as there were other personal issues which were contributing to this. She had been prescribed antidepressants.

Endoscopic evaluation of the larynx showed full abduction and adduction of the vocal folds with complete vocal fold closure. There was lateral constriction of the false vocal folds throughout but this was more prominent during the spoken sentences section of the endoscopic protocol. (see Figure 7.4a). Therapy techniques were trialled attempting to release the false vocal fold constriction. The silent giggle technique (see Figure 7.4b), humming, and accent method were all successful in releasing constriction and improving vocal quality. In particular it was noted that the degree of roughness quality reduced but her voice was not, however, within normal limits.

Case 5

Nicola, aged 27, was a primary school teacher working with reception children. She had a very heavy speaking and singing vocal load, as well as needing her voice at home looking after her five year old daughter. She had been teaching for two years and been experiencing vocal problems for six months before attending the voice clinic. She found that her voice would improve during the weekend and school holidays but by the end of the working week she could lose it completely. Although she reported feeling stressed by coping with her work/life bal-

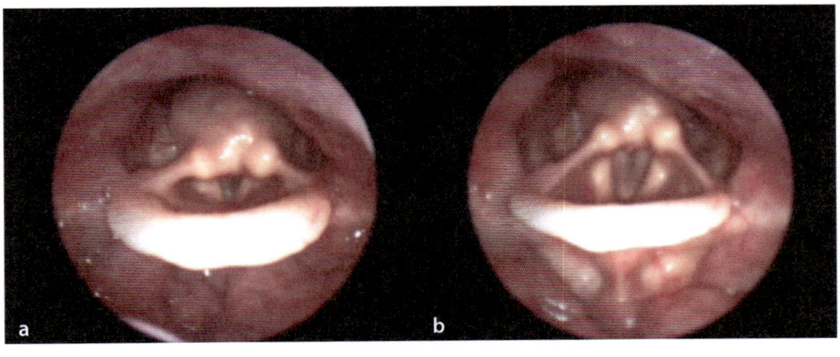

Figure 7.4: Kathleen. **a.** Lateral constriction of the false vocal folds. **b.** Silent giggle technique.

ance, she enjoyed teaching. She scored 20/40 on the Voice Handicap Index-10 and 34/40 on the Singing Voice Handicap Index-10.

When Nicola attended the voice clinic it was the end of the school holidays and she described her voice as better than usual. Her voice sounded mildly breathy and scored G1 R0 B1 A0 S0 on the GRBAS scale. Endoscopic evaluation showed the presence of very early vocal fold nodules with a moderate posterior glottic gap on phonation (see Figure 7.5a). When asked to imitate the dysphonia she produced a breathy, rough vocal quality with marked antero-posterior constriction (see Figure 7.5b). Nicola felt that this voice quality was consistent with how her voice sounded at the end of the working week. It is therefore reasonable to assume that this was the habitual vocal gesture she was producing as her voice deteriorated. It is likely that this constriction at supraglottic level was a result of her compensating for the inability to close her vocal folds along the full length. When asked to produce the twang gesture in section 7 of the protocol (Chapter 3) she did narrow the aryepiglottic sphincter but did not approximate the vocal folds, maintaining her breathy quality, resulting in an inability to project her voice.

The above case presentations illustrate the benefits of using endoscopic evaluation of the larynx as part of an assessment of the voce. The information gained helps to guide the voice therapist in the choice of appropriate techniques and helps the patient understand the benefits of therapy by providing visual feedback.

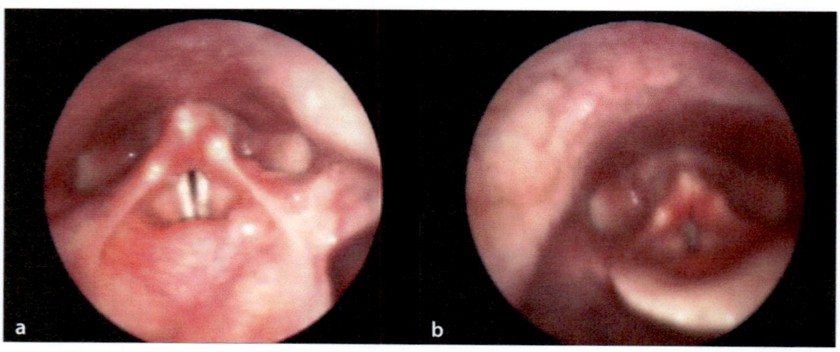

Figure 7.5: Nicola. **a.** Early vocal fold nodules with moderate posterior glottic gap on phonation. **b.** Imitated dysphonia showing antero-posterior constriction.

Bibliography

1. Harris, T., Harris, S., Rubin, J.S. and Howard, D.M. (eds) (1998) *The Voice Clinic Handbook*. London: Whurr Publishers Ltd.
2. Karnell, M. (1994) *Videoendoscopy: From Velopharynx to Larynx*. San Diego: Singular Publishing Group.
3. American Speech–Language–Hearing Association (1998) *The Roles of Otolaryngologists and Speech-Language Pathologists in the Performance and Interpretation of Strobovideolaryngoscopy*.
4. American Speech-Language-Hearing Association (2003) *Knowledge and Skills for Speech-Language Pathologists with Respect to Vocal Tract Visualization and Imaging*.
5. Carding, P.N., Jones, S.M., Morton, V., Robinson, F., Slade, S. and Wells, C. (2008) *Speech and Language Therapy Endoscopy for Voice Disordered Patients*. Position Paper 2008. Royal College of Speech and Language Therapists.
6. Harris, S. (1998) 'Speech therapy for dysphonia'. In Harris, T., Harris, S., Rubin, J.S. and Howard, D.M. (eds) *The Voice Clinic Handbook*, London: Whurr Publishers Ltd, pp. 139–206.
7. Colton, R. and Casper, J. (1990) *Understanding Voice Problems*. Baltimore, MD: Williams & Wilkins.
8. Mathieson, L. (2001) *The Voice and Its Disorders*. Sixth Edition. London: Whurr Publishers Ltd.
9. Sapienza, C. and Ruddy, B. (2009) *Voice Disorders*. San Diego, CA: Plural Publishing Inc.
10. Koschkee, D. and Rammage, L. (1997) *Voice Care in the Medical Setting*. San Diego, CA: Singular Publishing Group.
11. Rubin, J.S., Sataloff, R.T. and Korovin, G. (2014) *Diagnosis and Treatment of Voice Disorders*. Fourth Edition. San Diego, CA: Plural Publishing Inc.
12. Belafsky, P.C., Postma, G.N. and Koufman, J.A. (2002) 'Validity and reliability of the reflux symptom index (RSI)'. *J Voice*, **16**, 274–77. doi:10.1016/S0892-1997(02)00097-8
13. Belafsky, P.C., Postma, G.N. and Koufman, J.A. (2001) 'The validity and reliability of the reflux finding score (RFS)'. *Laryngoscope*, **111**, 1313–17. doi:10.1097/00005537-200108000-00001
14. Madill, C., Sheard, C. and Heard, R. (2010) 'Differentiated vocal tract control and the reliability of interpretations of nasendoscopic assessment'. *J Voice*, **24**, 337–45. doi:10.1016/j.jvoice.2008.09.008
15. Hirano, M. (1982) *Clinical Examination of Voice*. Vienna/New York, NY: Springer-Verlag.
16. Dejonckere, P.H., Obbens, C., de Moor, G.M. and Wieneke, G.H. 'Perceptual evaluation of dysphonia: reliability and relevance'. *Folia Phoniatr*, **45**, 76–83. doi:10.1159/000266220
17. Webb, A.L., Carding, P.N., Deary, I.J., MacKenzie, K., Steen, N. and Wilson, J.A. (2004) 'The reliability of three perceptual evaluation scales for dysphonia'. *Eur Arch Oto-Rhino-Laryngology*, **261**, 429–34. doi:10.1007/s00405-003-0707-7

18. Buckmire, R.A., Bryson, P.C. and Patel, M.R. (2011) 'Type I gore-tex laryngoplasty for glottic incompetence in mobile vocal folds'. *J Voice*, **25**, 288–92. doi:10.1016/j.jvoice.2009.12.003
19. Neuenschwander, M.C., Sataloff, R.T., Abaza, M.M., Hawkshaw, M.J., Reiter, D. and Spiegel, J.R. (2001) 'Management of vocal fold scar with autologous fat implantation: perceptual results'. *J Voice*, **15**, 295–304. doi:10.1016/S0892-1997(01)00031-5
20. Damrose, E.J. (2010) 'Percutaneous injection laryngoplasty in the management of acute vocal fold paralysis'. *Laryngoscope*, **120**, 1582–90. doi:10.1002/lary.21028
21. Tezcaner, C.Z., Ozgursoy, S.K., Sati, I. and Dursun, G. (2009) 'Changes after voice therapy in objective and subjective voice measurements of pediatric patients with vocal nodules'. *Eur Arch Oto-Rhino-Laryngology*, **266**, 1923–27. doi: 10.1007/s00405-009-1008-6
22. Akin Şenkal, Ö & Çiyiltepe, M. (2013) 'Effects of voice therapy in school-age children'. *J Voice*, **27**, 787. doi:10.1016/j.jvoice.2013.06.007
23. McCrory, E. (2001) 'Voice therapy outcomes in vocal fold nodules: a retrospective audit'. *Int J Lang Commun Disord*, **36**(Suppl), 19–24. doi:10.3109/13682820109177852
24. Lu, F.-L., Presley, S. and Lammers, B. (2013) 'Efficacy of intensive phonatory-respiratory treatment (LSVT) for presbyphonia: two case reports'. *J Voice*, 27, 786. doi:10.1016/j.jvoice.2013.06.006
25. Topaloğlu, İ., Koçak, I., Saltürk, Z. (2011) 'Multidimensional evaluation of vocal function after supracricoid laryngectomy with cricohyoidopexy'. *Ann Otol Rhinol Laryngol*, **121**, 407–12. doi:10.1177/000348941212100608
26. Kazi, R., Kiverniti, E., Prasad, V., Venkitaraman, R., Nutting, C.M., Clarke, P., *et al.* (2006) 'Multidimensional assessment of female tracheoesophageal prosthetic speech'. *Clin Otolaryngol*, **31**, 511–17. doi:10.1111/j.1365-2273.2006.01290.x
27. Yelken, K., Gultekin, E., Guven, M., Eyibilen, A. and Aladag, I. (2010) 'Impairment of voice quality in paradoxical vocal fold motion dysfunction'. *J Voice*, **24**, 724–27. doi:10.1016/j.jvoice.2009.05.004
28. Dejonckere, P.H., Remacle, M., Fresnel-Elbaz, E., Woisard, V., Crevier-Buchman, L. and Millet, B. (1996) 'Differentiated perceptual evaluation of pathological voice quality: reliability and correlations with acoustic measurements'. *Revue de laryngologie–otologie–rhinologie*, **177**, 219–24.
29. Langeveld, T.P.M., Drost, H.A., Zwinderman, A.H., Frijns, J.H.M. and Baatenburg De Jong, R.J. (2000) 'Perceptual characteristics of adductor spasmodic dysphonia'. Ann Otol Rhinol Laryngol, **109**, 741–48. doi:10.1177/000348940010900808
30. Carding, P., Carlson, E., Epstein, R., Mathieson, L. and Shewell, C. (2000) 'Formal perceptual evaluation of voice quality in the United Kingdom'. *Logoped Phoniatr Vocol*, **25**, 133–38. doi:10.1080/14015430050175860

31. Jones, S.M. and Carding, P.N. (2005) *Auditory perceptual evaluation of the voice: making progress*. Bulletin 10. Royal College of Speech and Language Therapists.
32. Jones, S.M. and Carding, P.N. (2006) *Roll out the GRBAS perceptual analysis scheme*. Bulletin 9. Royal College of Speech and Language Therapists.
33. Kempster, G.B., Gerratt, B.R., Abbott, K.V., Barkmeier-Kraemer, J. and Hillman, R.E. (2009) 'Consensus auditory-perceptual evaluation of voice: Development of a standardized clinical protocol'. *American Journal of Speech-Language Pathology*, **18**, 124–32. doi:10.1044/1058-0360(2008/08-0017)
34. Shewell, C. (2009) *Voice Work: Art and Science in Clinical Care*. Chichester, UK: Wiley-Blackwell.
35. Lieberman, J. (1998) 'Principles and techniques of manual therapy'. In Harris, T., Harris, S., Rubin, J.S. and Howard, D.M. (eds) *The Voice Clinic Handbook*, London: Whurr Publishers Ltd, pp. 91–138.
36. Chapman, J. (2011) *Singing and Teaching Singing: A Holistic Approach to Classical Voice*. Second Edition. San Diego, CA: Plural Publishing Inc.
37. Mathieson, L., Hirani, S.P., Epstein, R., Baken, R.J., Wood, G. and Rubin, J.S.. (2009) 'Laryngeal manual therapy: a preliminary study to examine its treatment effects in the management of muscle tension dysphonia'. *J Voice*, **23**, 353–66. doi:10.1016/j.jvoice.2007.10.002
38. Roy, N., Bless, D.M., Heisey, D. and Ford, C.N. (1997) 'Manual circumlaryngeal therapy for functional dysphonia: an evaluation of short- and long-term treatment outcomes'. *J Voice*, **11**, 321–31. doi:10.1016/S0892-1997(97)80011-2
39. Mathieson, L. (2011) 'The evidence for laryngeal manual therapies in the treatment of muscle tension dysphonia'. *Curr Opin Otolaryngol Head Neck Surg*, **19**, 171–76. doi: 10.1097/MOO.0b013e3283448f6c
40. Fawcus, M. (ed) (1991) *Voice Disorders and their Management*. New York, NY: Springer.
41. Jacobson, B.H., Johnson, A., Grywalski, C., Silbergleit, A., Jacobson, G., Benninger, M.S., *et al.* (1997) 'The Voice Handicap Index (VHI): Development and Validation'. *Am J Speech-Language Pathol*, **6**, 66–69. doi:10.1044/1058-0360.0603.66
42. Rosen, C.A., Lee, A.S., Osborne, J., Zullo, T., Murry, T. (2004) 'Development and validation of the voice handicap index-10'. *Laryngoscope*, **114**, 1549–56. doi:10.1097/00005537-200409000-00009
43. Cohen, S.M., Jacobson, B.H., Garrett, C.G., Noordzij, J.P., Stewart, M.G., Attia, A., *et al.* (2007) 'Creation and validation of the singing voice handicap index'. *Ann Otol Rhinol Laryngol*, 116, 402–6. doi:10.1177/000348940711600602
44. Deary, I.J., Wilson, J.A., Carding, P.N. and MacKenzie, K. (2003) 'VoiSS: A patient-derived Voice Symptom Scale'. *J Psychosom Res*, **54**, 483–89. doi:10.1016/S0022-3999(02)00469-5
45. Carding, P.N. (2000) *Evaluating Voice Therapy: Measuring the Effectiveness of Treatment*. London: Whurr Publishers Ltd.
46. Cohen, S.M., Statham, M., Rosen, C.A. and Zullo, T. (2009) 'Development and validation of the Singing Voice Handicap-10'. *Laryngoscope*, **119**, 1864–69. doi:10.1002/lary.20580

47. Ricci-Maccarini, A., De Maio, V., Murry, T. and Schindler, A. (2013) 'Development and validation of the children's voice handicap index-10 (CVHI-10)'. *J Voice*, **27**, 258. doi:10.1016/j.jvoice.2012.10.006

48. Epstein, R., Hirani, S.P., Stygall, J. and Newman, S.P. (2009) 'How do individuals cope with voice disorders? Introducing the Voice Disability Coping Questionnaire'. *J Voice*, **23**, 209–17. doi:10.1016/j.jvoice.2007.09.001

49. Hogikyan, N.D. and Sethuraman, G. (1999) 'Validation of an instrument to measure voice-related quality of life (V-RQOL)'. *J Voice*, **13**, 557–69. doi:10.1016/S0892-1997(99)80010-1

50. Jones, S.M., Carding, P.N. and Drinnan, M.J. (2006) 'Exploring the relationship between severity of dysphonia and voice-related quality of life'. *Clin Otolaryngol*, **31**, 411–17. doi:10.1111/j.1749-4486.2006.01291.x

51. Baken, R.J. (1987) *Clinical Measurement of Speech and Voice*. London: College-Hill Press.

52. Harris, T. (1998) 'Laryngeal mechanisms in normal function and dysfunction'. In Harris, T., Harris, S., Rubin, J.S. and Howard, D.M. (eds) *The Voice Clinic Handbook*, London: Whurr Publishers Ltd, pp. 64–87.

53. Harris, T. (1998) 'Vocal fold: structural and ultrastructural considerations for phonosurgeons'. in Harris, T., Harris, S., Rubin, J.S. and Howard, D.M. (eds) *The Voice Clinic Handbook*, London: Whurr Publishers Ltd, pp. 31–39.

54. *Control of Substances Hazardous to Health* [Internet]. Available from: http://www.hse.gov.uk/coshh/ [Accessed June 2015].

55. Weir, N. (1990) *Otolaryngology: An Illustrated History*. London: Butterworth & Company.

56. Schröck, A., Stuhrmann, N. and Schade, G. (2008) 'Flexible "chip-on-the-tip" endoscopy for larynx diagnostics'. *HNO*, **56**, 1239–42. doi: 10.1007/s00106-008-1783-1

57. Woo, P., Colton, R., Casper, J.K. and David, B. (1991) 'Diagnostic value of stroboscopic examination in hoarse patients'. *J Voice*, **5**, 231–38. doi:10.1016/S0892-1997(05)80191-2

58. Van Lierde, K.M., Claeys, S., De Bodt, M. and Van Cauwenberge, P. (2004) 'Outcome of laryngeal and velopharyngeal biofeedback treatment in children and young adults: a pilot study'. *J Voice*, **18**, 97–106. doi:10.1016/j.jvoice.2002.09.001

59. Bastian, R.W. and Nagorsky, M.J. (1987) 'Laryngeal image biofeedback'. *Laryngoscope*, **97**, 1346–49. doi:10.1288/00005537-198711000-00019

60. D'Antonio, L., Lotz, W., Chait, D. and Netsell, R. (1987) 'Perceptual-physiologic approach to evaluation and treatment of dysphonia'. *Ann Otol Rhinol Laryngol*, **96**, 187–90. doi:10.1177/000348948709600210

61. Maryn, Y., De Bodt, M. and Van Cauwenberge, P. (2006) 'Effects of biofeedback in phonatory disorders and phonatory performance: A systematic literature review'. *Applied Psychophysiology Biofeedback*, **31**, 5–83. doi:10.1007/s10484-006-9005-7

62. McFarlane, S. and Lavorato, A. (1984) 'The use of video endoscopy in the evaluation and treatment of dysphonia'. *Commun Disord*, **9**, 117–26.

63. Rattenbury, H.J., Carding, P.N. and Finn, P. (2004) 'Evaluating the effectiveness and efficiency of voice therapy using transnasal flexible laryngoscopy: a randomized controlled trial'. *J Voice*, **18**, 522–33. doi:10.1016/j.jvoice.2004.01.003

64. Piazza, C., Del Bon, F., Peretti, G. and Nicolai, P. (2012) 'Narrow band imaging in endoscopic evaluation of the larynx'. *Curr Opin Otolaryngol Head Neck Surg*, **20**, 472–76. doi:10.1097/MOO.0b013e32835908ac

65. Švec, J.G. and Schutte, H.K. (1996) 'Videokymography: High-speed line scanning of vocal fold vibration'. *J Voice*, **10**, 201–5. doi:10.1016/S0892-1997(96)80047-6

66. Kendall, K.A. (2012) 'High-speed digital imaging of the larynx: recent advances'. *Curr Opin Otolaryngol Head Neck Surg*, **20**, 466–71. doi:10.1097/MOO.0b013e328359840d

67. Laeeq, K., Pandian, V., Skinner, M., Masood, H., Stewart, C.M., Weatherly, R., *et al.* (2010) 'Learning curve for competency in flexible laryngoscopy'. *Laryngoscope,* **120**, 1950–53. doi:10.1002/lary.21063

68. Sunkaraneni, V.S. and Jones, S.E. (2011) 'Topical anaesthetic or vasoconstrictor preparations for flexible fibre-optic nasal pharyngoscopy and laryngoscopy'. *Cochrane Database Syst Rev*, **16**, CD005606. doi:10.1002/14651858.CD005606.pub2

69. Koufman, J. (2014) 'Evaluation of laryngeal biomechanics by transnasal flexible laryngoscopy'. In Rubin, J.S., Sataloff, R.T. and Korovin, G.,(eds) *Diagnosis and Treatment of Voice Disorders*, fourth edition. San Diego, CA: Plural Publishing Inc., pp. 223–33.

70. Frosh, A.C., Jayaraj, S., Porter, G. and Almeyda, J. (1998) 'Is local anaesthesia actually beneficial in flexible fibre-optic nasendoscopy?' *Clin Otolaryngol Allied Sci*, **23**, 259–62. doi:10.1046/j.1365-2273.1998.00149.x

71. Sadek, S.A.A., De, R., Scott, A., White, A.P., Wilson, P.S. and Carlin, W.V. (2001) 'The efficacy of topical anaesthesia in flexible nasendoscopy: A double-blind randomised controlled trial'. *Clin Otolaryngol Allied Sci*, **26**, 25–28. doi:10.1046/j.1365-2273.2001.00400.x

72. Smith, J.C. and Rockley, T.J. (2002) "A comparison of cocaine and "co-phenylcaine" local anaesthesia in flexible nasendoscopy'. *Clin Otolaryngol Allied Sci*, 27, 192–96. doi:10.1046/j.1365-2273.2002.00563.x

73. Cain, A.J., Murray, D.P. and McClymont, L.G. (2002) 'The use of topical nasal anaesthesia before flexible nasendoscopy: A double-blind, randomized controlled trial comparing cophenylcaine with placebo'. *Clin Otolaryngol Allied Sci*, **27**, 485–88.

74. Johnson, P.E., Belafs, P.C. and Postma, G.N. (2003) 'Topical nasal anesthesia for transnasal fiberoptic laryngoscopy: a prospective, double-blind, cross-over study'. *Otolaryngol - Head Neck Surg*, **128**, 452–54. doi:10.1016/S0194-5998(02)23294-5

75. Georgalas, C., Sandhu, G., Frosh, A. and Xenellis, J. (2005) 'Cophenylcaine spray vs. placebo in flexible nasendoscopy: A prospective double-blind randomised controlled trial'. *Int J Clin Pract*, **59**, 130–33. doi:10.1111/j.1742-1241.2005.00476.x

76. Douglas, R., Hawke, L. and Wormald, P.J. (2006) 'Topical anaesthesia before nasendoscopy: a randomized controlled trial of co-phenylcaine compared with lignocaine'. *Clin Otolaryngol*, **31**, 33–35. doi:10.1111/j.1749-4486.2006.01129.x

77. Bourolias, C., Gkotsis, A., Kontaxakis, A. and Tsoukarelis, P. (2010) 'Lidocaine spray vs tetracaine solution for transnasal fiber-optic laryngoscopy'. *Am J Otolaryngol*, **31**, 114–16. doi: doi:10.1016/j.amjoto.2008.11.011

78. Shrestha, B. and Amatya, R. (2013) 'Local anesthesia versus placebo in flexible nasopharyngo-laryngoscopy'. *J Rhinolaryngo-Otologies*, **1**, 52–56. doi:10.12970/2308-7978.2013.01.01.10

79. Mahrous, A., Tysome, J. and Davis, J. (2012) 'A prospective randomised controlled trial in one hundred and eleven patients to determine whether flexible nasendoscopic laryngosocpy is more comfortable for patients when performed above or belwo the inferior turbinate'. *Clin Otolaryngol*, **37**, 223–44. doi:10.1111/j.1749-4486.2012.02483.x

80. Hu, A., Moore, J.E., Rose, B., Fort, S., Gracely, E.J. and Sataloff, R.T. (2014) 'The effect of oral topical anesthesia on the characteristics of voice'. *J Voice*, **28**, 92–97. doi:10.1016/j.jvoice.2013.07.011

81. Jacobs, M.A. and Kenny, D.T. (2005) 'Effects of topical anesthetic and flexible fibre-optic laryngoscopy on professional sopranos'. *J Voice*, **19**, 645–64. doi:10.1016/j.jvoice.2004.10.002

82. Pothier, D.D., Raghava, N., Monteiro, P. and Awad, Z. (2006) 'A randomized controlled trial: Is water better than a standard lubricant in nasendoscopy?' *Clin Otolaryngol*, **31**, 134–37. doi:10.1111/j.1749-4486.2006.01173.x

83. *Patient Group Directions in the NHS* [Internet]. Available from: http://www.mhra.gov.uk/Howweregulate/Medicines/AvailabilityprescribingsellingandsupplyingofmedicinesExemptionsfromMedicinesActrestrictions/PatientGroupDirectionsintheNHS/index.htm [Accessed June 2015]

84. Carding, P.N., Jones, S., Morton, V., Robinson, F., Slade, S. and Wells, C. (2008) *Speech and Language Therapy Endoscopy for Voice Disordered Patients*. RCSLT position paper 2008.

85. Sataloff, R.,Hawkshaw, M., Sataloff, J.B., DeFatta, R.A. and Eller, R. (2012) *Atlas of Laryngoscopy*. Third edition. San Diego, CA: Plural Publishing Inc.

86. Woo, P. (2010) *Stroboscopy*. San Diego, CA: Plural Publishing Inc.

87. Morrison, M. and Rammage, L. (1994) *The Management of Voice Disorders*. London: Chapman & Hall Medical.

88. Havas, T. and Priestley, J. (1993) 'The revised Australian fiberscopic profile'. *J Voice*, **7**, 377–81. doi:10.1016/S0892-1997(05)80261-9

89. Williams, R.S., Lancaster, J., Karagama, Y., Tandon, S. and Karkanevatos, A. (2004) 'A systematic approach to the nasendoscopic examination of the larynx and pharynx'. *Clin Otolaryngol Allied Sci*, **29**, 175–78. doi:10.1111/j.0307-7772.2004.00784.x

90. Singh, A. and Lyons, M. (2004) 'Minimum dataset for the recording of findings of flexible nasopharyngolaryngoscopy'. *J Laryngol Otol*, **118**, 972–73. doi:10.1258/0022215042790655

91. Hirano, M. and Bless, D.M. (1993) *Videostroboscopic Examination of the Larynx*. San Diego, CA: Whurr Publishers Ltd.

92. Poburka, B.J. (1999) 'A new stroboscopy rating form'. *J Voice*, **13**, 403–13. doi:10.1016/S0892-1997(99)80045-9

93. Johnson, I.J., Carding, P.N., Heywood, S. and Relf, G.T. (1996) 'Vocim–a system for measuring the larynx endoscopically'. *Clin Otolaryngol Allied Sci*, **21**, 308–11. doi:10.1111/j.1365-2273.1996.tb01076.x

94. Brewer, D. and McCall, G. (1974) 'Visible laryngeal changes during voice therapy: fiber-optic study'. *Ann Otol Rhinol Laryngol*, **83**, 423–27.

95. Stemple, J., Glaze, L. and Klaben, B. (2010) *Clinical Voice Pathology: Theory and Management*. Fourth edition. San Diego CA: Plural Publishing Inc.

96. Colton, R. and Estill, J. (1981) 'Elements of Voice Quality: Perceptual, Acoustic and Physiologic Aspects'. In Lass, N. (ed) *Speech and Language: Advances in Basic Research and Practice*, San Diego, CA: Academic Press, pp. 311–404.

97. Estill, J. and McDonald Klimek, M. (2005) *Primer of Compulsory Figures: Level Two: Figure Combinations for Six Voice Qualities*. Santa Rosa, CA: Estill Voice Training Systems International.

98. Sundberg, J. (1989) *The Science of the Singing Voice*. DeKalb, IL: Northern Illinois University Press.

99. Titze, I.R. (2000) *Principles of Voice Production*. Second edition. Iowa City, IA: National Center for Voice and Speech.

100. Titze, I.R. and Verdolini Abbott, K. (2012). *Vocology: The Science and Practice of Voice Habilitation*. Iowa City, IA: National Center for Speech and Voice.

101. Estill, J. (1992) *Basic Figures and Exercise Manual*. New York, NY: Imagetech.

102. Chalfin, D. and Jones, S.M. (2010) 'Endoscopic assessment of dysphonic singers: a new model'. British Voice Association, Choice for Voice Conference.

103. McDonald Klimek, M. and Estill, J. (2005) *Estill Voice Training System; Primer of Compulsory Figures: Level One. Compulsory Figures for Voice Control*. Santa Rosa, CA: Estill Voice Training Systems International.

104. Boone, D., McFarlane, S., Von Berg, S. and Zraick, R. (2014) *The Voice and Voice Therapy*. Ninth Edition. Pearson.

105. Sataloff, R.T., Hawkshaw, M.J., Divi, V. and Heman-Ackah, Y.D. (2007) 'Physical examination of voice professionals'. *Otolaryngol Clin North Am*, **40**,953–69. doi:10.1016/j.otc.2007.05.004

106. Bless, D.M., Hirano, M. and Feder, R.J. (1987) 'Videostroboscopic evaluation of the larynx'. *Ear Nose Throat*, **66**, 289–96.

107. Miller, M.K. and Verdolini, K. (1995) 'Frequency and risk factors for voice problems in teachers of singing and control subjects'. *J Voice*, **9**, 348–62. doi:10.1016/S0892-1997(05)80197-3

108. Elias, M.E., Sataloff, R.T., Rosen, D.C., Heuer, R.J. and Spiegel, J.R. (1997) 'Normal strobovideolaryngoscopy: Variability in healthy singers'. *J Voice*, **11**, 104–7. doi:10.1016/S0892-1997(97)80030-6

109. Lundy, D.S., Casiano, R.R., Sullivan, P.A., Roy, S., Xue, J.W. and Evans, J. (1999) 'Incidence of abnormal laryngeal findings in asymptomatic singing students'. *Otolaryngol - Head Neck Surg*, **121**, 69–77. doi:10.1016/S0194-5998(99)70128-2

110. Phyland, D.J., Oates, J. and Greenwood, K.M. (1999) 'Self-reported voice problems among three groups of professional singers'. *J Voice*, **13**,:602–11 doi:10.1016/S0892-1997(99)80014-9

111. Sataloff, R.T. (2005) *Professional Voice: The Science and Art of Clinical Care*. Third edition. San Diego, CA: Plural Publishing Inc.

112. Harris, D. (1998) 'Singing and therapy'. In Harris, T., Harris, S., Rubin, J.S. and Howard, D.M. (eds) *The Voice Clinic Handbook*, London: Whurr Publishers Ltd, pp. 207–45.

113. Chagnon, F., Hassan, S. and Purdy, W. (1998) 'The mechanics of messa di voce'. *La Scena Musicale*, **4**(4).

114. Kayes, G. (2004) *Singing and the Actor*. Second edition. London: A&C Black.

115. Sadolin, C. (2012) *Complete Vocal Technique*. Third edition. Copenhagen: CVI Publications.

116. McGlashan, J., Sadolin, C. and Kjelin, H. (2008) 'Can vocal effects such distortion, growling, rattle and grunting be produced without traumatising the vocal folds'. Queen's Medical Centre, Nottingham, UK.

117. Koufman, J.A., Radomski, T.A., Joharji, G.M., Russell, G.B. and Pillsbury, D.C. (1996) 'Laryngeal biomechanics of the singing voice'. *Otolaryngol - Head Neck Surg*, **115**, 527–37. doi:10.1016/S0194-5998(05)80592-3

118. Belafsky, P.C., Postma, G.N., Reulbach, T.R., Holland, B.W. and Koufman, J.A. (2002) 'Muscle tension dysphonia as a sign of underlying glottal insufficiency'. *Otolaryngol - Head Neck Surg*, **127**, 448–51. doi:10.1067/mhn.2002.128894

119. Verdolini, K., Rosen, C. and Branski, R. (2006) *Classification Manual for Voice Disorders*. New York, NY: Psychology Press.

120. Morrison, M.D., Rammage, L.A. (1993) 'Muscle misuse voice disorders: description and classification'. *Acta Otolaryngol*, **113**, 428–34. doi: 10.3109/00016489309135839

121. McGlashan, J., Costello, D. and Bradley, P.J. (2007) 'Hoarseness and voice problems'. In Ludman, H. and Bradley, P.J. (eds) *ABC of Ear, Nose and Throat*. Fifth edition. Oxford: BMJ Books, pp. 71–77.

122. Koufman, J. (1995) 'Evaluation of laryngeal biomechanics by fibre-optic laryngoscopy'. In Rubin, J.S., Sataloff, R.T., Korovin, G. and Gould, W.J. (eds) *Diagnosis and Treatment of Voice Disorders*. San Diego, CA: Igaku-Shoin, pp. 122–34.
123. Baker, J. (1998) 'Psychogenic dysphonia: peeling back the layers'. *J Voice*, **12**, 527–35. doi:10.1016/S0892-1997(98)80061-1
124. Butcher, P., Elias, A. and Cavalli, L. (2007) *Understanding and Treating Psychogenic Voice Disorder: A CBT Framework*. Chichester, UK: John Wiley & Sons Ltd.
125. Murphy, A. (1964) *Functional Voice Disorders*. New Jersey: Prentice-Hall Inc.
126. Boone, D. (1977) *The Voice and Voice Therapy*. Second edition. New Jersey: Prentice-Hall Inc.
127. Stemple, J., Glaze, L. and Klaben, B. (2010) *Clinical Voice Pathology: Theory and Management*. Fourth edition. San Diego, CA: Plural Publishing Inc.
128. Behrman, A. and Haskell, J. (2013) *Exercises for Voice Therapy*. Second edition. San Diego, CA: Plural Publishing Inc.
129. Casper, J.K. and Murray, T. (2000) 'Voice therapy methods in dysphonia'. *Otolaryngol Clin North Am*, **33**, 983–1002. doi:10.1016/S0030-6665(05)70259-0
130. Prater, R. (1991) 'Voice therapy: techniques and applications'. *Otolaryngol Clin North Am*, **24**, 1075–92.
131. Prater, R. and Swift, R. (1984) *Manual of Voice Therapy*. Texas: Pro-Ed Inc.
132. Thyme, K. and Frokjaer-Jensen, B. (2001) *The Accent Method: A Rational Voice Therapy in Theory and Practice*. Bicester, UK: Speechmark.
133. McDonald Klimek, M. and Estill, J. (2005) *Estill Voice Training System; Primer of Compulsory Figures: Level One. Compulsory Figures for Voice Control*. Santa Rosa, CA: Estill Voice Training Systems International.
134. Bagnall, A.D. (1992) *The Complete Voicecraft Manual*. Adelaide, Australia: Voice International.
135. Verdolini-Abbot, K. (2008) *Lessac-Madsen Resonant Voice Therapy*. San Diego, CA: Plural Publishing Inc.
136. Pichler, K. (2005) 'The Lee Silverman Voice Treatment (LSVT): An evidence based voice and speech treatment for individuals with Parkinson's disease'. *Nervenheilkunde* [Internet], **24**, 873.
137. Dejonckere, P.H. and Lebacq, J. (2001) 'Plasticity of voice quality: a prognostic factor for outcome of voice therapy?' *J Voice*, **15**, 251–56. doi:10.1016/S0892-1997(01)00025-X
138. Carding, P.N., Horsley, I.A. and Docherty, G.J. (1999) 'A study of the effectiveness of voice therapy in the treatment of 45 patients with nonorganic dysphonia'. *J Voice*, **13**, 72–104. doi:10.1016/S0892-1997(99)80063-0
139. Carding, P.N. and Horsley, I.A. (1992) 'An evaluation study of voice therapy in non-organic dysphonia'. *Eur J Disord Commun*, **27**, 137–58. doi:10.3109/13682829209012036

140. Gartner-Schmidt, J.L., Roth, D.F., Zullo, T.G. and Rosen, C.A. (2013) 'Quantifying component parts of indirect and direct voice therapy related to different voice disorders'. *J Voice*, **27**, 210–16. doi:10.1016/j.jvoice.2012.11.007

141. Nasser Kotby, M. and Fex, B. (1998) 'The Accent Method: Behavior readjustment voice therapy'. *Logopedics Phoniatrics Vocology*, **23**, 39–43. doi:10.1080/140154398434329

142. Coblenzer, H. and Muhar, F. (1976) *Atem und Stimme: Anleitung zum guten Sprechen*. Munich: Österreichischer Bundesverlag.

143. Boone, D.R. and McFarlane, S.C. (1993) 'A critical view of the yawn-sigh as a voice therapy technique'. *J Voice*, **7**, 75–80. doi:10.1016/S0892-1997(05)80114-6

144. Guzman, M., Castro, C., Testart, A., Muñoz, D. and Gerhard, J. (2013) 'Laryngeal and pharyngeal activity during semioccluded vocal tract postures in subjects diagnosed with hyperfunctional dysphonia'. *J Voice*, **27**, 709–16. doi:10.1016/j.jvoice.2013.05.007

Index

About the Authors

Sue M. Jones, BSc., MSc., RCSLT

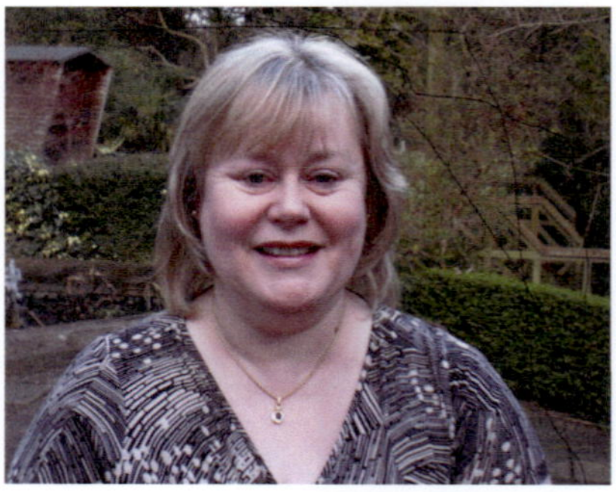

Sue Jones is Head of Speech, Voice and Swallowing Services at University Hospital of South Manchester, UK. Sue has specialised in Clinical Voice Disorders since 1984 and now works exclusively in this field. She has been instrumental in developing the voice clinic services at UHSM and now acts and as an Expert Advisor, Speech and Language Therapy, where she leads a team of voice specialists, in performing, interpreting and teaching laryngeal endoscopy.

Her particular interests are in developing competencies for practice in all aspects of voice disorders: from newly qualified, to expert level therapists. Sue carried out research into the relationship between severity of dysphonia and voice-related quality of life as part of a Masters Clinical Research programme at Newcastle University. This has led to further interest in and study of the perceptual analysis of voice disorders.

Sue also has a particular interest in the performing voice and has developed her skills in working with professional singers, including classical, musical theatre and rock and pop genres. Her work here led to the establishment of a specialist Performers Voice Clinic service at UHSM.

An adviser to the Royal College of Speech and Language Therapists on voice disorders and co-author of the RCSLT Position Paper on Endoscopy for Voice Disordered Patients, Sue has lectured nationally and internationally and is involved in leading and participating in a variety of research projects into voice disorders.

Carrie Garrett, BA (Hons) Music/Popular Music, BSc (Hons) Speech and Language Therapy, PGCE, cert., MRCSLT, HCPC

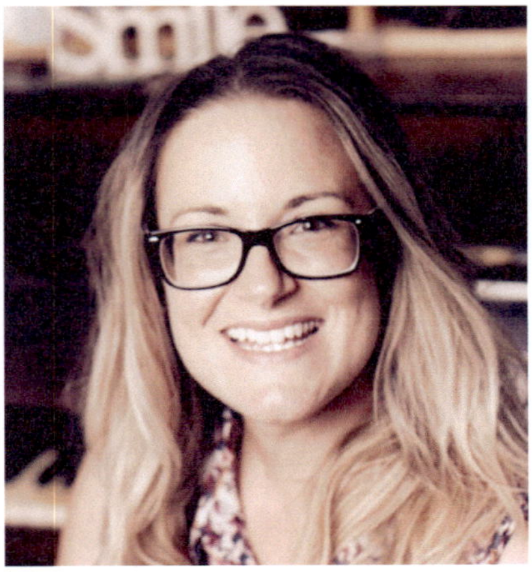

Carrie is a voice specialist, speech and language therapist and singing teacher. Her clinical work includes working as a voice specialist at Queen Elizabeth Hospital, Birmingham, UK, and as singing-voice rehabilitation specialist at University Hospital South Manchester, where she has been working closely with Sue Jones and others in the development of the protocol contained in this publication.

Aside from regular appearances as a live performer, she is a singing teacher with 18 years experience, having also run a vocational education music performance department for a number of years. In addition to her work as a Voice Therapist, she runs her own vocal tuition company.

Printed by Libri Plureos GmbH in Hamburg,
Germany

9 781909 082199